What Everyone Can Do to

# Fight
# AIDS

# What Everyone Can Do to

# Fight
# AIDS

ANNE GARWOOD *&* BEN MELNICK

Jossey-Bass Publishers
San Francisco

Substantial discounts on bulk quantities of Jossey-Bass books are available to
corporations, professional associations, and other organizations. For details and
discount information, contact the special sales department at Jossey-Bass Inc., Publishers,
(415) 433-1740; Fax (415) 433-0499.

For international orders, please contact your local Paramount Publishing
International office.

 Manufactured in the United States of America on Lyons Falls Pathfinder
Tradebook. This paper is acid-free and 100 percent totally chlorine-free.

LIBRARY OF CONGRESS CATALOGING-IN-PUBLICATION DATA

Garwood, Anne, date.
    What everyone can do to fight AIDS : a primer for families and
friends / Anne Garwood, Ben Melnick.
        p.     cm.
    ISBN 0-7879-0044-3
    1. AIDS (Disease)—Popular works.    1. Melnick, Ben, date.
11. Title.
RC607. A26G375       1995                                    94-37646
362. 1'969792—dc20

FIRST EDITION
*PB Printing*  10  9  8  7  6  5  4  3  2  1

# Contents

# Acknowledgments

The authors gratefully acknowledge Alan Rinzler and Susan Garwood for all their advice and support. And many thanks to Dr. Molly Cook of San Francisco for checking the medical facts in this book.

*To Craig and Nick*
*and all those whose lives*
*have been touched*
*by HIV and AIDS*

# Foreword

At this point, in our society, almost everyone has lost someone to AIDS. We grieve the loss and we wonder at the senselessness of it all. We often want to take action and fight back, yet too often we stop because we simply don't know where to begin. The disease is bigger than us all and we feel helpless in its shadow.

My message to you is simply this: we can illuminate that darkness, one step at a time. One day at a time. One neighborhood at a time. One community at a time.

This book, *What Everyone Can Do to Fight AIDS*, will teach you how. The AIDS epidemic affects us all. Likewise, this book addresses us all—everyone who wants and needs to know about AIDS: men, women, children . . . entire families.

You will learn the facts and dispel the myths. You will learn what to do and what not to do. Hopefully, you will be inspired to get involved, on whatever level works for you. Every single act counts, no matter how big or small. You do make a difference.

*What Everyone Can Do to Fight AIDS* is both a source of vital information and a call for action. Please join me in the commitment to fight this dreadful epidemic. Together, we must make a difference.

ELTON JOHN

# Introduction

There are many reasons why you might be reading this book. Perhaps you are curious about the AIDS epidemic or concerned for your family's safety. Maybe you need ways to protect yourself and your children, or you want tips on how to become more involved in the fight against AIDS. Perhaps AIDS threatens a loved one or a member of your family, maybe even yourself.

The AIDS epidemic is a great tragedy, but there is much cause for hope. Although there is no cure yet, AIDS is completely preventable. Education and smart choices can stop the spread of the disease. As more effective treatment is developed, people are living longer. Those who once were afraid of or hateful toward people with AIDS are now beginning to understand their need for support and compassion. Also, individuals from a wide variety of communities are recognizing the importance of learning about HIV and AIDS and are helping others to learn as well.

2

So let's learn more about it, do everything we can to prevent it, and—even more—join the effort against it in any way we can, large or small.

This book will help us to confront our fears with the most important, specific, and up-to-date information available and answer questions such as:

* What is AIDS?
* How does it spread?
* What is the difference between being HIV positive and having AIDS?
* How can I protect my family from AIDS?
* What should I tell my children about AIDS?
* How should I act around someone who is HIV positive or has AIDS?
* What are the latest medical strategies to fight AIDS?

Once we have a greater understanding of what AIDS is, the book will go on to explore other important topics such as:

* What can I do to provide emotional support?
* How can I help in my own community?
* What can young people do about AIDS?
* Which organizations can best use my services?
* What other kinds of social or political action would be appropriate?

This book offers both information and inspiration. It provides the basic facts about AIDS, suggests where to go for more information, and offers tips and ideas about ways to become involved in the fight against the disease. Reading this book can be an important first step for you and your family to take in learning about AIDS.

# Learning About HIV and AIDS

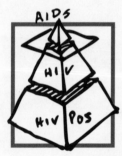

In spite of the confusing and sometimes conflicting information you may have pieced together from newspapers, magazines, friends, and television shows, it's easy to learn the basic facts about how AIDS spreads and why it is deadly. This chapter provides the essential facts about HIV—human immunodeficiency virus—and AIDS and lists resources to help you learn more about the AIDS epidemic.

# What is AIDS?

AIDS stands for acquired immunodeficiency syndrome—a fatal disorder of the immune system. A person with AIDS gradually loses the ability to fight off infections and cancers that would ordinarily be stopped by the immune system. Conditions that are not serious for normally healthy people, such as the common cold or flu, can be very severe for people with AIDS and can lead to the further weakening of their immune systems. People living with AIDS also become especially vulnerable to specific diseases, called opportunistic infections, which range from moderately dangerous to deadly. These infections, not AIDS itself, ultimately cause death. The initial cause of immune system breakdown is infection with HIV.

## What causes AIDS?

AIDS is caused by a virus named the human immuno-deficiency virus (HIV). When someone is infected with HIV, the virus invades cells, called T-cells or helper cells, which are important components of the immune system. T-cells help orchestrate the immune system's response to conditions that threaten the body.

HIV multiplies inside T-cells, eventually killing them entirely. As more and more cells die, the immune system is less able to do its job. Infected people have a more difficult time fighting off germs and are highly susceptible to common colds or flus. Gradually, as their systems are weakened by constant battle with germs we normally would repel every day, they develop rare and unusually severe infections; these infections usually lead to the diagnosis of full-blown AIDS. The infections may attack in many ways, sometimes targeting the respiratory and sensory systems and, in some cases, even brain function, eventually shutting these organs and systems down.

HIV does not immediately weaken a person's immune system. It can take as much as ten years or more or as little as a few months after infection for HIV to seriously damage the immune system. The length of time between initial infection and full-blown AIDS depends on many factors, such as a person's lifestyle, attitude, and body chemistry.

## *What is the history of AIDS?*

Early in 1981, physicians and medical researchers in
the United States began to notice a rare type of cancer,
called Kaposi's sarcoma (or KS), appearing in homosexual
men. Many of these men also seemed to suffer from an
immune suppression that left them vulnerable to infections, some of which had never been diagnosed in humans
before. Many of these patients were dying from a virulent
form of pneumonia, called Pneumocystis carinii pneumonia, which is common only to those with impaired
immune systems.

As the search for the origins of this strange new
malady began, some disturbing trends began to appear.
Hemophiliacs and recipients of blood transfusions began
to exhibit similar symptoms of immune suppression.
Intravenous drug users also began dying terrible and inex-
plicable deaths from Pneumocystis pneumonia. An
increasing number of babies were born with inadequate
immune systems and were quickly dying. It became
apparent that all of these deaths were related to this mys-
terious new problem, and that the problem was not one
solely for the gay community.

Unfortunately, the association of this new disease with
homosexuals brought up many conflicting feelings. Since

gays were not widely accepted by mainstream society in the United States, early efforts to begin research into causes and to provide clinical support for those afflicted were not a high priority. Because no one understood how the disease was spread, there was widespread confusion and panic; those living with the disease were stigmatized. Hysteria about AIDS transmission combined with fears about homosexuality to create a fierce backlash against gays and against efforts to fight AIDS. Many medical researchers believe that this backlash, along with the federal government's inaction, hampered strong preventative education efforts and led to the needless infection of thousands of people. According to Randy Shilts in his best-selling book *And the Band Played On*, embarrassment prevented a strong and unified public response. AIDS was ". . . about sex, and it was about homosexuals. Taken altogether, it had simply embarrassed people—the politicians, the reporters, the scientists. AIDS had embarrassed everyone . . . and tens of thousands of Americans would die because of that" (page 582).

Scientists suspected from the beginning that they were dealing with a bloodborne virus—one that was passed in much the same way hepatitis is passed, through the exchange of blood and semen. It took a long time to prove this fact and to isolate the virus that causes AIDS.

During this time, blood banks could not adequately test their supplies for the virus, and the federal government did not get involved in a significant way. In testimony before subcommittee hearings on AIDS in August of 1983, Marcus Conant, a San Francisco dermatologist with an ever-growing load of Kaposi's sarcoma cases, said of the government's response to AIDS: "The failure to respond to this epidemic now borders on a national scandal. Congress, and indeed the American people, have been misled about the response. We have been led to believe that the response has been timely and that the response has been appropriate, and I would suggest to you that that is not correct" (*And the Band Played On*, p. 359).

Meanwhile, people were dying. There had been more than 12,000 reported cases in the United States by mid 1985, and of these, more than 6,000 people had died. The early response to the epidemic in the United States was centered in the gay community. Most of the AIDS service organizations in existence today were created and sustained by gays, lesbians, and their families and friends. During the years when no one in power seemed to be paying attention to AIDS, it was the dedicated—and angry—members of this group who fought for more funding and greater compassion from the government and the public at large.

## PANDEMIC: WHEN AN EPIDEMIC IS WORLDWIDE

In December 1994, the San Francisco Chronicle reported that there had been 401,749 AIDS cases and 243,423 deaths from AIDS in the United States as of mid 1994.

Worldwide, the numbers are staggering. According to the World Health Organization, 17 million people have been infected with HIV, and an estimated 4 million people have developed AIDS. And AIDS continues its terrible reign. Experts now predict that by the year 2000, 12 to 14 million people will have AIDS worldwide. In 1994, the Center for International Research of the U.S. Bureau of the Census projected that by the year 2010, AIDS will have a major impact on life expectancy in many nations. In Thailand, life expectancy will be cut by thirty years; in Zambia it will be cut in half.

### THE GROWTH OF HIV INFECTION, WORLDWIDE

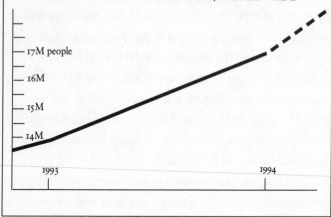

It took the announcement, in 1985, that film star Rock Hudson had been stricken with AIDS to make the country take real notice of the disease. Once the news broke, AIDS entered the public consciousness in a whole new way. While support and funding still lagged behind, more people were getting the message that AIDS is a terrible disease that requires compassion and a massive effort of education.

During the 1980s, the United States was not the only country struggling with the disease. It was one of the only places, however, where AIDS was viewed as a primarily gay disease. In Africa, it was known as "slim disease," because of the wasting and weight loss it typically caused, and was spreading primarily in the heterosexual community. Today, the AIDS epidemic is really a global pandemic that touches lives on every continent and affects all kinds of people across the world.

## *How is AIDS spread?*

--------------

HIV is actually quite delicate and can only be spread in specific and favorable conditions. Although the virus is found in trace amounts in other bodily fluids and tissues, it is in highest concentration in blood, semen, vaginal secretions, and breast milk. Any practice in which an infected person and a noninfected person might exchange these fluids has the potential to spread the virus. Having unprotected sex (sex without condoms) and sharing needles to inject drugs are the most common activities that spread AIDS.

Since the virus is so delicate, it cannot be spread by:

* Making casual contact (shaking hands, patting on the back, routine touching)
* Hugging an infected person
* Drinking from the glass an infected person has used
* Sitting on a toilet seat an infected person has used
* Being at work or at school with someone who is HIV positive
* Being bitten by a mosquito

There are many ways to protect yourself against the virus. Chapter Two will discuss how HIV is spread and which practices are safe or dangerous.

# Who can get AIDS?

In the early days of the epidemic, homosexual men were the first to show the effects of AIDS. Because of this, people associated AIDS with gays and assumed that heterosexuals were not at risk. This mistaken notion persists today, even as heterosexual men, women, and even small children and the elderly are dying from this disease. Although AIDS was first seen in the gay community, it is not a picky virus. It does not discriminate on the basis of gender, skin color or sexual orientation. AIDS is an equal-opportunity killer.

People who are getting AIDS include:

* Those who practice unsafe sex, whether they are gay or straight, single or married; whether they do it all the time or "just this once"
* People who use needles to inject drugs (including steroids) and share dirty needles with other users
* Babies born to infected mothers

Although many people have died as a result of receiving infected blood during a transfusion, blood and blood products have been tested for HIV since 1985, and the blood supply is now safe. Hemophiliacs, who depend on blood products to stop the uncontrollable bleeding common to their condition, were especially hard hit. Since the necessary clotting agents are now tested, new infections among hemophiliacs are much less likely today.

14

## *How can people tell if they have been infected with HIV?*

- - - - - - - - - - -

Since HIV can be present for many years without causing any noticeable symptoms, the only way to know for sure if you are HIV positive is to be tested by a health care professional. The test itself is just a simple blood draw, like many other medical procedures; the hard part is coping with your feelings. While you wait for two weeks to get your results, you may have many worries:

※ What if I am HIV positive?

※ Will people find out that I have been tested?

※ How will my life change if the news is bad?

※ Do I really want to know?

※ Why do I have to deal with this?

These feelings are very common and nothing to be ashamed about. Most testing centers offer valuable counseling services before and after testing to help relieve some of the anxiety associated with testing and to answer any questions you may have.

Getting tested forces you to confront the possibility that you might have to deal with AIDS in a very personal way. It's not easy, but it's important. If you are HIV positive, getting early treatment can mean years of additional life. Getting tested is also the only responsible way to fully protect those with whom you are intimate. It's a good idea to be tested every six months if you have been exposed to any risk factors. Sometimes HIV infection does not show up in tests for up to six months after exposure.

Because of the stigma surrounding HIV infection, many people are hesitant to come forward and be tested. To help alleviate the fear of public exposure, therefore, anonymous testing is widely available and is the best way to ensure that a test result remains confidential. At a test site that offers this service, you never give your name. Instead, you are assigned a number and the only way to get your test result is in person, using that number. This ensures that your result will be confidential.

16

## What is the difference between being HIV positive and having AIDS?

AIDS is the condition caused by HIV. People do not catch AIDS—they are exposed to the virus that causes AIDS, HIV. People with HIV usually appear healthy and some show no signs of sickness for many years. A doctor diagnoses a patient with clinical or full-blown AIDS when HIV has weakened the immune system to the extent that certain diseases or infections known as opportunistic infections appear. Even if no opportunistic infections are present, a doctor may also diagnose AIDS when an HIV-infected person's T-cell count falls below a certain level, usually 200 cells per cubic milliliter or less. For the average healthy person, a T-cell count of 480 to 1,800 is normal. Although AIDS is the term most commonly used to describe the final stages of HIV infection, many people have begun to use the term "HIV disease" to refer to all the phases of HIV infection, from initial seroconversion (production of antibodies) to full-blown AIDS.

# *What are the symptoms of AIDS?*

AIDS symptoms are the result of the opportunistic infections that take advantage of a weakened immune system. These infections produce the most noticeable symptoms commonly associated with AIDS. Two people with AIDS may have very different symptoms, depending on which infections they have.

The initial HIV infection often produces ordinary cold and flu symptoms such as fatigue, mild fever, and tender lymph glands. These symptoms usually go away in a week or two, and a silent phase begins. This silent phase often masks a gradual progression of damage to the immune system over a period of several months to many years.

At some point, symptoms due to HIV may develop—a stage of the disease sometimes called AIDS–related complex (ARC). At one time, experts believed that ARC was a different condition caused by HIV that was related to but not the same as AIDS. Today, the consensus is that ARC is merely a condition of progression toward full-blown AIDS.

When the silent phase ends, a range of subtle, then progressively more severe symptoms appears. An infected person may experience fatigue, lymph node swelling or tenderness, night sweats, weight loss, chronic diarrhea, mouth and tongue infections, ear-nose-throat problems, a fall in platelet count (blood cell fragments that help in clotting), or skin disease. A person at this stage of the disease can experience many ups and downs, both physically and emotionally. Some who are able to stabilize their health through changes in lifestyle, diet, and medical treatment live in relatively good health for many years. Others deteriorate rapidly. The more we learn about AIDS and about sickness in general the more we realize how important having a hopeful and life-affirming attitude is to the healing process.

In the final, or clinical, stages of AIDS, people have many symptoms of immune deficiency, including weight loss (hence the name wasting syndrome) and a falling T-cell count. They often have several severe opportunistic infections at the same time. Their condition may fluctuate dramatically from day to day, even hour to hour, a process that has been compared to a long roller-coaster ride with many highs and lows.

Several opportunistic infections (see opposite) are common to the advanced stages of AIDS. Many of these infections can be treated individually with varying degrees of success, but each infection leaves the immune system in a more weakened state, making it easier for the next infection to cause even greater damage.

## OPPORTUNISTIC INFECTIONS

CRYPTOCOCCAL MENINGITIS: a condition caused by a fungus that infects the brain and spinal cord—may cause headache, confusion, fever, blurred vision, and speech difficulties and can lead to coma and death

CYTOMEGALOVIRUS (CMV): a virus that can cause blindness, encephalitis, pneumonia, and gastrointestinal disorders

DEMENTIA: an impairment of brain function that can be caused by subacute encephalitis, by a low-grade infection of the brain, or by atrophy of the brain's tissues

HISTOPLASMOSIS: a condition characterized by widespread tissue infection and chronic fever

KAPOSI'S SARCOMA: a type of skin cancer characterized by painless pink or purplish lesions and found most commonly in gay men with AIDS

LYMPHOMAS: cancer of the lymph glands that may develop while the T-cell count is still normal

PNEUMOCYSTIS CARINII PNEUMONIA (PCP): a special form of pneumonia that is usually treatable but which may cause permanent lung damage

SHINGLES: painful blisters that itch underneath the skin and are caused by a reactivation of the chicken pox virus

THRUSH: a yeast-like fungus infection of the mouth—often one of the first signs of a weakened immune system

TOXOPLASMOSIS: a microscopic parasite that can be found in raw or undercooked meat or cat feces—can lead to seizures, brain inflammation, coma, and death

TUBERCULOSIS: an infectious disease that is commonly considered to be a lung problem but which can affect any part of the body

Several infections, cancers, and other conditions combine to weaken and ultimately kill people with AIDS, but many of these conditions are treatable, especially if detected early. The earlier HIV is found and symptoms are treated, the less damage is done to the immune system and the longer the life span. As the epidemic continues, health care professionals are learning how to manage opportunistic diseases more effectively, and people with AIDS are living longer.

# *How is AIDS treated medically?*

Medical treatment for HIV infection and AIDS is of two types: antiviral treatment, which is aimed at slowing the spread of the virus within the body, and treatments that are specialized for each of the opportunistic infections. For an HIV-positive person who does not yet have opportunistic infections, antiviral treatment is the focus. If caught early enough, HIV infection and its progress toward AIDS, and eventually death, can be slowed.

Unfortunately, none of the antiviral treatments used against HIV are sufficiently effective, and some have severe side effects. The most common antiviral treatment is azidothymidine (AZT), one of the only drugs currently licensed by the U.S. government for treatment of HIV infection. AZT does not kill the virus, but it blocks the enzyme that the virus uses to reproduce itself, thus slowing the progress of the disease.

People taking AZT often experience fatigue, headaches, nausea, muscle aches, insomnia, fevers, and rashes. AZT also interferes with bone marrow function, which in turn causes anemia. Many people cannot tolerate these side effects. Scientists have also found that HIV can become resistant to AZT.

Other promising antiviral drugs are available that may prove to be less toxic for some users. These drugs are designed to work alone or in concert with AZT. Some doctors have combined these and other treatments in varying amounts to form "cocktails" that are mixed to suit the needs of particular patients. These treatments have had some success in slowing the progress of the disease.

While no antiviral drug can completely stop the spread of AIDS in the body, many individualized treatments can help alleviate the symptoms of the various opportunistic diseases. These treatments are as diverse as the diseases they are designed to fight. Many offer relief to a patient whose immune system may not be strong enough to fight off a predatory infection.

### The patient–physician relationship

The patient-physician relationship is also an important consideration in treating AIDS. Since AIDS is a unique disease that is not yet fully understood, treatment options vary widely from patient to patient and from symptom to symptom. Since AIDS is apparently almost always fatal, many who live with it feel they have nothing to lose—and everything to gain—by pursuing an aggressive and some-times experimental course of treatment.

Many people with AIDS have kept up with the latest research and developments in treatment so they can play an informed role in their own health care. A number of them have participated in trials of new drugs and other treatments. People with AIDS have also played a major role in agitating for a faster review process for new drugs by the Food and Drug Administration (FDA) and for increased government funding for AIDS research, services, and education. This has led to a shift in the balance of power between doctor and patient, prompting physicians to be more responsive and respectful of their patients' treatment ideas and more willing to experiment with new drugs and alternative therapies. The patient can be his or her own best advocate.

## 24

# *How does lifestyle affect the treatment of AIDS?*

Many people living with AIDS have significantly improved their health by changing their lifestyle and becoming actively involved in their own health care. Although there has not been adequate clinical study in this area, most experts and AIDS patients believe that a number of controllable "cofactors" play a significant role in halting the progress of AIDS. People living with AIDS have reported strengthening their immune systems by improving their diets, exercising moderately, stopping smoking, drinking less (or no) alcohol, abstaining from recreational drugs, getting plenty of rest, avoiding stress, and generally cultivating habits that would be beneficial to anyone. A healthy lifestyle is important to everyone's health, but it is vital to those with weakened immune systems.

One of the most important factors in staying well with HIV infection is nutrition. A balanced diet, eaten in good

> "All the alternative treatments, at the very least, are directed toward creating the attitudes that enhance healing; and many people find that various of the alternatives have worked for them ... to create active healing."—ALAN I. HAMILL, *The AIDS Caregiver's Handbook*, p. 76.

amounts, can make a real difference to the health of people who are HIV positive and particularly those with full-blown AIDS. As AIDS progresses and people begin to lose a lot of weight, their bodies become debilitated to the point of starvation. Without abundant nutrients, the body's already weakened immune system has no way to recover; opportunistic infections have free reign, and death is hastened.

A significant number of people with AIDS have found various types of alternative and traditional medicine to be helpful, particularly those practices that provide nurturing and attentive care to individuals. Some of the popular forms of alternative treatment include:

* Acupuncture
* Affirmation techniques
* Body work
* Creative visualization
* Herbal medicine
* Homeopathy
* Massage
* Meditation
* Support groups
* Vitamin therapy

Many of these approaches are especially effective in reducing stress, which most experts agree is important in maintaining the strength of the immune system. Alternative health care also emphasizes maintaining the strong and hopeful attitude that is so vital for living longer with AIDS.

## Spiritual practice

Many people with AIDS turn to some type of spiritual practice for solace. Religious groups can provide support and inspiration to those facing crisis. Many churches have joined together to form the AIDS Interfaith Network, which is designed to offer pastoral support and counseling to those with AIDS and their loved ones. Some strengthen their current practice or turn to the religion of their youth; others find strength through the many AIDS interfaith network healing services and groups. Some turn to other practices, such as Buddhism or other eastern religions. Whether formal or informal, alone or in groups, spiritual practice offers hope to those who might not otherwise find it, helps foster a positive attitude, and again, helps reduce stress. These factors play a subtle but tremendously important role in the health of people with AIDS.

## *What about a cure?*

- - - - - - - - - - - -

According to experts at the 1993 International
Conference on AIDS, there is no cure in sight. But
researchers are making progress. As more is learned and
treatments are improved, people with AIDS are living
longer. And a great deal of promising research is under-
way, even though scientists have just begun to understand
how HIV works to cause AIDS.

Immunologists are optimistic about the eventual development of a vaccine, but there are a tremendous number
of obstacles to the testing and marketing of such a product. The virus that causes AIDS constantly mutates and
changes, making it difficult to isolate a strain that would
be useful in developing a vaccine. Some work has been
done using portions of the virus that do not change.
These vaccines have shown promise in laboratory animals,
but no animal develops AIDS after infection with HIV, so
these results may not be meaningful in humans. Tests with
human volunteers are also very difficult. Since it is not
possible to expose people to HIV after they have been
vaccinated, the only way to find out if the vaccine is effective is to test a large number of people and monitor them
for years to see if their infection rate is lower than that of
unvaccinated people.

All experts agree that the best—indeed, the only—way to fight AIDS now is with massive educational efforts to stop the spread of HIV, especially in young people. For those who are already living with HIV and AIDS, compassionate care and access to the latest treatments should be available, along with support and information about alternative treatments and about how to live a healthy lifestyle.

In the next chapter we will discuss in greater detail how to prevent the spread of AIDS.

# LEARNING MORE ABOUT HIV AND AIDS

At the end of most of the chapters in this book, there is a list of resources—books, audiotapes, videotapes, or other references—to help you learn more about the ideas discussed in the chapter. A listing of HIV- and AIDS-related organizations appears at the back of this book.

### General books about HIV and AIDS

*AIDS: The Facts* by JOHN LANGONE (Little, Brown, 1991)

*The AIDS Reader: Social, Political and Ethical Issues* by NANCY MCKENZIE (Meridian Books, 1991)

*Living with AIDS* edited by STEPHEN R. GRAUBARD (MIT Press, 1991)

*The Social Impact of AIDS in the United States* edited by ALBERT R. JONSEN and JEFF STRYKER (National Academy Press, 1993)

### Books about the history of AIDS

*And the Band Played On: Politics, People and the AIDS Epidemic* by RANDY SHILTS (Penguin Books, 1988)

*As Real as It Gets: The Life of a Hospital at the Center of the AIDS Epidemic* by CAROL POGASH (Plume, 1992)

*Bearing Witness: Gay Men's Health Crisis and the Politics of AIDS* by PHILIP M. KAYAL (Westview Press, 1993)

*The Search for the Virus: The Scientific Discovery of AIDS and the Quest for a Cure* by STEVE CONNOR and SHARON KINGMAN (Penguin Books, 1989)

30

### Books about AIDS as a global issue

*AIDS in the World: A Global Report* edited by JONATHAN MANN, DANIEL J. M. TARANTOLA and THOMAS W. NETTER (Harvard University Press, 1992)

### Books about AIDS and alternative health care

*Healing AIDS Naturally* by LAURENCE E. BADGELEY (Human Energy Press, 1987)

*Surviving with AIDS: A Comprehensive Program of Nutrition Co-Therapy* by C. WAYNE CALLAWAY (Little, Brown, 1991)

# Preventing AIDS

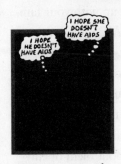

While there is still no cure, we have a big advantage in the fight against AIDS. Unlike many other deadly diseases—such as cancer—we know how HIV spreads and how to prevent its transmission. For the informed person, AIDS is a completely preventable disease. With effective education and prevention programs, we can stop the spread of the disease.

The best way to help yourself and your loved ones avoid AIDS is by being open about the risky behaviors that can lead to infection with HIV. Talking about AIDS means talking about sex and drugs and other topics that may be uncomfortable for you. You may disapprove of them; you may not want to bring them up with your family or face them yourself. In the age of AIDS, however, open and accepting dialogue about risks and choices is a must. It is vital that everyone—young, old, and in-between—knows how the virus that causes AIDS is transmitted. Discussing risky practices does not mean that you have to approve of them. In fact, you can make your views known more clearly by talking about them openly rather than by remaining silent.

Young people today face more risks than their parents did. They need to meet these risks with complete knowledge not only so they can avoid danger but so they won't have unnecessary fear or treat others with prejudice.

This chapter discusses how AIDS is spread—which behaviors are safe and which are risky—and what you can do to protect yourself and minimize the risk.

# *How the AIDS virus is spread*

The good news is that the virus that causes AIDS is actually very fragile. It can't live outside the body, and it's very picky about the conditions under which it will spread from one person to another. Unless the fluids or tissues in which it is concentrated are directly exchanged, it dies of exposure soon after it leaves the body. Most experts agree that HIV cannot survive outside the body for longer than thirty minutes. The majority of cases of HIV infection result from the exchange of blood or semen. Other fluids in which the virus lives are not easily exchangeable.

There are really only a few ways to catch the virus. These include:

### Vaginal sex

Vaginal sex (when a man penetrates a woman's vagina with his penis) is the most commonly practiced form of sex for heterosexuals. If a man is infected with HIV, the fluids from his penis can introduce the virus into the woman's bloodstream through tiny tears in the lining of the vagina.

### Anal sex

Anal sex (when a man penetrates the anus of his sex partner with his penis) is the most risky type of sex. The

34    rectum (the passage inside the anus) is lined with delicate blood vessels that bleed easily during sex. This makes it even easier for fluid from an infected man's penis to enter the bloodstream of his sex partner. Some experts believe it is also possible for HIV to directly infect cells lining the rectum.

### Oral sex

The virus can also be passed by licking or sucking a partner's genitals or anus. Fluids can enter the bloodstream through sores or invisible cuts in the mouth, which are almost always present (think about what happens when you floss your teeth or eat a piece of toast). Experts are not sure if the AIDS virus can enter the bloodstream through the digestive tract when semen is swallowed.

### Sharing needles

Sharing needles to inject drugs is one of the most common ways HIV is spread. Injecting drugs is a very dangerous practice in its own right. If you or a friend or loved one are injecting drugs, you need to get help from a drug treatment program. When a syringe is used by a person infected with the virus, a small amount of their blood is drawn back up into the needle. If the same needle is then used by another person without being properly sterilized, the infected blood enters that person's bloodstream.

### *From mother to child*

One-third of the babies born to women infected with HIV are infected themselves. The virus can be passed from mother to child through the placenta. It can also be transmitted during birth in vaginal secretions and blood or through breast milk.

### *Blood exchange rituals*

Many teenagers participate in some type of blood exchange ritual to seal a friendship, become "blood brothers," or show membership in a gang. HIV can easily be transmitted in this way. There is no safe way to become blood brothers.

### *Blood transfusions*

Before testing of the blood supply began in the United States in 1985, a number of people were infected with the virus by receiving transfusions of infected blood. Currently, all blood supplies are thoroughly tested, so there is little chance of infection from receiving blood.

36

## Avoiding risk

By now you should have a good sense of what constitutes dangerous behavior. And what is unsafe sex or drug use tonight is even more dangerous than it was ten years ago because more people are HIV positive. In these risky times, you should make a lifetime commitment to taking good care of yourself. What, then, are the habits and precautions you should follow now that you understand the risks?

**To be safe, everyone must *identify, avoid, escape,* or *manage* high-risk situations.**

### Practicing abstinence

Abstinence means not having sex. Abstinence is the surest way to avoid contracting HIV, but it is very hard to practice in today's sexually charged environment. Movies, advertisements, television, and popular music all constantly use sex to sell themselves. Young people, and even many adults, consider it normal to begin having sex in early adolescence. Young people themselves often feel sex is an important step to maturity; most adults think it is essential to a romantic and intimate relationship.

Given all this, abstinence can be a tough sell. No one likes to feel out of it or uncool, but not having sex does not mean that you're a prude or that you can't touch and be sensual. It also doesn't mean that you can't be close to anyone or be romantically involved. In the age of AIDS, hasty or impulsive sex is not the ideal way to initiate or sustain romantic involvement. Instead of just saying, "No," how about saying, "Let's wait"?

### Being monogamous

If you do choose to have a sexual relationship, monogamy greatly reduces the chance of contracting HIV. In a monogamous relationship, both partners have sex only with each other. If you and your partner never have sex with anyone else, and neither of you has the virus, there is little chance of infecting each other. You should still use a condom, however. Unless both of you have been tested and found to be free of HIV, condoms should still be used. The virus can be present for six months before showing up in a test, so you should be tested twice at six-month intervals to make sure you are not infected. Even then, you should not have sex without a condom unless you have complete trust that your partner is also monogamous. And that trust is tough to come by. Studies have shown that many people lie about their HIV status—when they know it—and that most people don't know their HIV status, which is even more dangerous.

### Using condoms

If you choose to have sex, using a condom properly can prevent infection because it prevents fluid from the penis from entering the vagina or anus. Be sure to use latex condoms. Other types, like sheepskin condoms, do not stop HIV. The man must put on a condom while his penis is erect but before any penetration; the condom won't form a seal if the penis is not erect. The fluid that comes out of the penis before ejaculation can contain HIV, so you or your partner should put on a condom before any penetration.

There are vaginal foams and creams containing the spermicide Nonoxynol 9 that kill HIV, but they should be used in addition to—and not instead of—a condom. A condom should be removed immediately after ejaculation. As the penis becomes less erect, the seal around the edges of the condom becomes less secure, and fluids may leak out. Never reuse a condom. If you are using a condom along with a sexual lubricant, make sure that the lubricant is water-based. Oil-based lubricant can dissolve latex.

During oral sex, be sure to use a condom or a dental dam. There are specially designed nonlubricated condoms for use in oral sex (many are flavored). Using a dental dam—a square piece of latex that is placed over the

## CONDOM LAWS

**L** Use LATEX condoms. Natural sheepskin condoms have pores that allow the virus to pass through.

**A** Make sure you have condoms AVAILABLE. (They don't work if you don't use them!)

**W** Always use WATER-BASED LUBRICANTS like K-Y Jelly. Vaseline and other petroleum-based lubricants will dissolve condoms.

**S** Use a SPERMICIDE like Nonoxynol 9. Condoms with spermicide added are much more effective. You can also put spermicidal gels inside the condom and inside the vagina or anus.

### ADDITIONAL TIPS

Store condoms in a COOL, DRY PLACE, not in your wallet or the glove box of your car, because heat will break down the latex.

Buy condoms MADE IN THE UNITED STATES because of the quality control laws. Glow-in-the-dark condoms from Taiwan are decorative but ineffective against HIV.

Check the EXPIRATION DATE on the package, and do not use the product if its expiration date has passed.

Make sure "FOR DISEASE PREVENTION" is on the label.

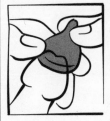 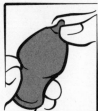 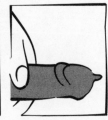

40

woman's genital region—prevents the exchange of fluid that might contain the AIDS virus. You can also use a condom that has been slit up the side to form a flat piece of latex.

### Avoiding drugs and alcohol

Using drugs and alcohol before sex is very risky. Drugs and alcohol often increase your desire for sex while reducing your judgment and reason. You are much more likely to have unsafe sex if you are intoxicated or high on drugs. Susan, an AIDS educator in Nebraska, says:

*"Alcohol and drugs don't just impair your judgment. They also make it physically difficult to be safe. Many people in the workshops I do aren't convinced until I do a demonstration. I have someone come to the front of the room, where I have a wrapped condom and a cucumber. First, I spin them around for sixty seconds and then I ask them to put the condom on the cucumber. Most people have trouble just getting the wrapper open."*

## KNOWING WHICH PRACTICES ARE RISKIEST

Some sexual practices are riskier than others. It's important to be careful, especially when you engage in higher-risk activities, such as anal or vaginal intercourse.

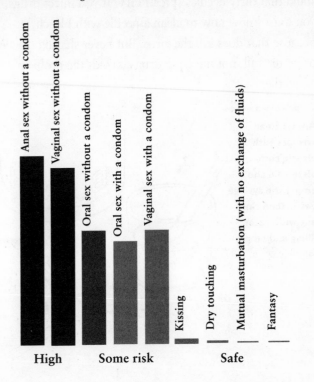

## 42 *Cleaning needles*

No one wants to encourage others to inject drugs, but if you do so, use a clean needle. Everyone needs to understand that dirty needles spread HIV. If you inject drugs, you must know how to clean a needle with bleach, because that does kill the virus. But never sharing needles, or better still, not injecting drugs, avoids the problem altogether.

Always clean syringes with bleach; completely fill and empty the syringe twice, then rinse out with water, filling and emptying twice.

# Common questions about HIV infection

Even though we understand how the virus that causes AIDS usually spreads, some people may still have questions about particular situations and practices. If you understand the basic concepts that have been discussed already, the answers to these questions may be obvious, but you also may find them reassuring.

### Can I catch it from a toilet seat?

No. HIV dies outside the human body. It cannot live when exposed to the open air. It can only be exchanged if a fluid in which it is concentrated enters the bloodstream.

### Can I get it at work?

It is not possible to catch the virus from the type of contact most people have at work. You can only get it from the specific practices listed earlier in this chapter— mainly unsafe sex and sharing needles. If you do not do these things at work with your co-workers, you will not catch the virus at work.

### Could I get it from mosquitoes?

No. The virus dies and becomes harmless when it leaves the human body. It cannot survive in blood that has been drawn by a mosquito. Many studies have shown conclusively that mosquitoes cannot transmit HIV.

### Is kissing safe?

Kissing is probably safe. HIV has been found in small amounts in the saliva of some people, but researchers have never found AIDS to be spread by kissing. There isn't enough of the virus in saliva to cause infection. If an infected person with a cut or sore on the lips or mouth kisses another person with a cut in the mouth, it is theoretically possible for the virus to be passed in infected blood. But most scientists agree that you can enjoy kissing without worry.

### How about hugging and touching?

Hugging, touching, massaging, handshaking, and other forms of casual contact are completely safe. Human skin is very tough and is impermeable to germs and viruses. HIV is too large to pass through the skin, so unless the skin is broken by a cut or sore, there is no way for the virus to get through.

Touch is essential to our health, happiness, and well-being. We express a great deal of acceptance, reassurance, and affection in the ways we touch each other as we go about our business or spend time with friends and loved ones. People who don't know any better are sometimes physically afraid of people with AIDS and won't touch them, even if they show no signs of disease. People with AIDS sorely miss this type of contact.

### What about giving and getting blood?

There is no risk in giving blood. Blood donation facilities use only disposable needles, so there is no chance you can get the virus from a dirty needle while performing this important public service. Since 1985, all blood banks have tested their blood supplies, so there is almost no chance of receiving infected blood. If someone donates blood very soon after becoming infected, it is remotely possible that the virus would not show up when the blood is tested. If you know you will be needing blood in the future, you may want to ask your physician about drawing some of your own blood for storage.

# LEARNING MORE ABOUT HOW TO BE SAFE

### Books about being safe

*201 Things You Should Know About AIDS and Other Sexually Transmitted Diseases* by JEFFREY S. NEVID (Allyn & Bacon, 1993)

*Safe Sex in the Age of AIDS: For Men and Women* by the INSTITUTE FOR THE ADVANCED STUDY OF HUMAN SEXUALITY (Citadel Press, 1986)

### For brochures, pamphlets, and booklets about HIV and AIDS contact:

IMPACT AIDS INC.
3692 18th Street
San Francisco, CA 94110
415/ 861-3397

CENTER FOR HEALTH
INFORMATION
P.O. Box 4636
Foster City, CA 94404
415/345-6669

# Teaching Your Children

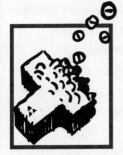

You may have heard the statistics: HIV is the fifth leading cause of death among young people. Twenty percent of all people diagnosed with AIDS were probably infected during their teenage years. Teens have among the fastest-growing rates of new HIV infection.

You know that teaching your children about AIDS is one of the most important, challenging, and necessary things you will do as a parent. You know that your children need vital information about HIV transmission that will help them make good choices and possibly save their lives. You know all of these things . . . and you also know that AIDS is a tough subject to talk about. It brings up uncomfortable issues like sex and sexuality, intravenous drug use, and death. How can you talk about these things with a young person? And how can you not?

In this chapter, ways of getting the vital message about HIV and AIDS to young people will be explored—ways that are appropriate to their age and comfortable for you as a parent. While AIDS is never a simple topic to bring up with children, several helpful suggestions and resources can make your task easier.

# Why talk to young children?

It is important to discuss AIDS with children before they become sexually active so they will have the knowledge and judgment they will need later on. While broaching the topic with teens may seem easier, younger children are usually more receptive to learning from parents and other authority figures. So it makes a lot of sense to begin the dialogue with your children when they are quite young.

For example, children who have been taught the value and importance of recycling from a very early age tend to make it a lifelong habit. Recycling becomes a part of who they are—separating paper and plastic is automatic. The same can be true of children who learn about HIV and AIDS at an early age. They will know how to be safe, and they will make choices that will help keep them safe throughout their lives.

There are many basic approaches to informing children about AIDS without alarming or traumatizing them. You can also make your message age-appropriate, telling your children as much as they need to know at their particular stage of life. If you are extremely uncomfortable bringing the topic up, you can use books, videos, or even other adults who know the facts and want to share them, such as the family doctor or scout troop leader. Many school clubs and organizations, AIDS service organizations, or even church youth groups have AIDS awareness materials and programs. The important thing is to make sure your child gets the message. Many of the tips offered in this chapter are useful for any age-group. Be sure to read through the suggestions for all the age-groups, whether or not your child fits that category.

## *Talking with children under eight years old*

AIDS is a part of virtually everyone's life. While your child may not know anyone who is infected, chances are that he or she has heard the term and probably some scary—perhaps incorrect—information along with it. The focus for children under eight is not on the specifics of HIV transmission or on how the virus affects the body. Instead, you should give them general information that dispels the frightening myths and rumors about AIDS. You should also encourage them to be compassionate and kind to people who are living with the disease. The following tips will help guide your efforts:

❋ BE CONCRETE. When talking to very young children, emphasize simple concepts and be careful not to frighten them or give them more information than they can handle.

❋ DON'T TALK DOWN. Your message will be more effective if you make sure not to talk down to children. Take them where they are, and answer their questions as openly as you can. Young people hate to feel as though they are too young, or as if they are being condescended or lectured to. If they sense that you do not take them seriously, they may feel reluctant to discuss the topic with you in the future.

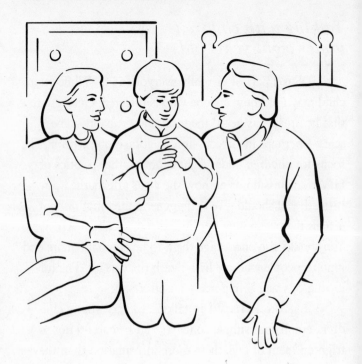

✳ ASK WHAT THEY KNOW. Ask what they have heard about AIDS already. They may have questions or fears based on wrong information. Younger children have a difficult time understanding the stigma that surrounds AIDS, so it is vital to emphasize that people with AIDS are just that—people—and that they deserve love and compassion and support.

✳ ACKNOWLEDGE THEIR FEARS. AIDS is a part of the culture. Children probably hear many mixed messages about AIDS that may frighten or confuse them. If your child asks you about AIDS, it is important to respond openly and avoid acting shocked or angry about their curiosity. If you appear upset or disturbed by the topic, this will discourage them from asking important questions about AIDS. It is important to build a relationship of trust when it comes to difficult subjects such as this.

**Some common questions young children may ask and suggested answers**

*What is AIDS?*

AIDS is a group of diseases that are caused by a virus called HIV. This virus can cause people to die because it affects the immune system, which is what keeps you healthy.

54

*How do you get AIDS?*

You get AIDS-related disease from HIV. People with HIV get it from other people who already have it.

*Will I get HIV?*

You will not get HIV because it's very difficult to get it from other people. The virus must go directly into your blood from someone else's blood and that's very hard to do. (Young children live in the here-and-now. Don't try to explain what might happen if they practice risky behaviors when they get older.)

*Why do some children have AIDS?*

Some people get HIV when they are born. If a mother has HIV, she can pass it into her child's bloodstream during pregnancy or birth. This didn't happen to you because I'm not infected with HIV.

Some other children have gotten the virus when they were sick and needed extra blood. A long time ago, some of the blood that doctors gave to their patients had the virus that causes AIDS in it, and so the virus went into the people along with the blood. This rarely happens now because doctors only give people blood that is tested for HIV; only blood that is free of the virus is used.

*Will I get HIV from a kid in my school who has it?*

No, you will not. HIV and AIDS are not passed to other people who live and play with infected people. You can play with infected children, swim in the same pool, use the same toilet and water fountain, or share the same toys, and you won't get HIV.

*Do people with AIDS get better?*

Right now, there is no cure for AIDS, but new medicines and treatments are helping people who have it stay healthy for many years.

## 56 *Talking to children aged eight to eleven*
- - - - - - - - - - - -

Children at this age are better able to understand abstract ideas such as viruses. This is the age to bring up how the virus that causes AIDS works in the body—how it progresses from HIV infection, to AIDS, to eventual death. This is also the age to begin discussing how people can protect themselves against HIV and AIDS and the importance of being safe. Most children are aware by this time that AIDS has something to do with sex and drugs. Specifically, you should:

✳ GIVE THEM THE FACTS. Present the simple facts about AIDS and HIV, using pictures of HIV invading T-cells. See the resources to help with this listed at the end of this chapter.

✳ TALK ABOUT CHOICES. While you may not want to go into great detail about safe sex and clean needles with this age group, it is important to emphasize that the presence of AIDS means that they must make important choices in the future and that these choices can mean life or death.

✳ PREPARE THEM WELL. Help to lay the groundwork for good choices by encouraging your child to be smart and by giving them the tools they will need.

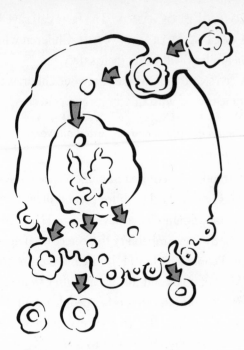

HIV-1 (top right) enters a T lymphocyte cell in the bloodstream. Usually, the T-cell identifies and destroys viral invaders, but HIV-1 is able to neutralize the T-cell and then use it to replicate itself. The T-cell becomes an HIV factory (a retrovirus) that will explode with hundreds more HIV-1 virions. These rapidly search for and invade other T-cells, effectively closing down the body's immune system.

58

Among the most important tools a child can acquire are:

* CORRECT INFORMATION. The facts can save lives.
* A GOOD SENSE OF SELF-WORTH. Children who value themselves will value their safety.
* A LISTENING EAR. Make sure your children can come to you with questions and concerns.

### More common questions and suggested answers

*What is AIDS?*

AIDS stands for acquired immunodeficiency syndrome. This is a medical term for certain illnesses caused by the human immunodeficiency virus or HIV. This virus stops the body's natural ability to protect itself against infections. People who have HIV are more prone to getting the kind of colds and flus we all suffer from. They also get serious illnesses that other people usually don't get, like rare cancers, infections, or pneumonia. These conditions eventually cause them to die.

*Do only gay people get AIDS?*

No. When AIDS first hit the news in the early 1980s, it seemed to be infecting only people in the gay community. Many nonhomosexual people thought they were safe from becoming infected. But that wasn't true. Now it is clear that anyone—men, women, children, husbands, wives,

grandfathers, ministers, teachers—anyone can become
infected with HIV.

*How do you get AIDS?*

AIDS is caused by a virus that passes from an infected
person to another person. But it's a different kind of virus
from the cold or flu viruses that people give to one another
when they sneeze or cough or hold hands. HIV passes
from one person to another only when blood or other
bodily fluids infected with HIV go from the infected person directly into the blood or body of another person.

If young people get HIV, they are usually infected in
one of two ways: they get the virus from their mothers or
from blood transfusions. Children can become infected
with HIV during their mother's pregnancy or at birth if
their mothers were already infected with HIV and the
virus passes into the bloodstream of the newborn child. It
is very rare, but HIV can be passed to an infant from an
infected mother through breast feeding. Some children
also become infected with HIV from medical blood transfusions that were given before 1985 when the blood supply
wasn't yet tested for HIV the way it is today.

Older people can get the virus in two other ways. One
way is by using HIV-infected needles to inject drugs into
their bodies. When a person with HIV uses a needle or
syringe to shoot drugs and then lets another person use it,

the infected blood that is still on the needle can be injected into the second person. Then that second person may develop HIV, too. Another way to get it is through unprotected sexual intercourse with a person who is infected with HIV.

*How can I tell if someone has HIV?*

You cannot tell by looking at someone whether he or she has HIV. In fact, people who have the virus may not know it themselves because they have no symptoms yet. People with AIDS only look sick when they develop cancers or infections that result from HIV infection.

*Can I get HIV from someone in my school who has it?*

No. No one has ever gotten HIV from another person through casual contact. HIV cannot go from one person to another the way a cold, the flu, or the chicken pox can—through coughing, sneezing, touching, or playing. HIV is not catching that way, so you can't get it by sharing toilets, pencils, desks, secrets, telephones, food, or doorknobs. In fact, children with HIV can play, eat, sleep, kiss, and fight with their brothers and sisters and their parents. There has never been a case of HIV transmission from this kind of day-to-day contact.

However, the HIV-infected child may endanger his or her health by playing with you. Because HIV weakens the body's ability to fight off illnesses, the child with HIV might easily catch your cold or flu virus and become very ill because that child's immune system is not as strong as it needs to be. But you have nothing to worry about. You will not get HIV from an infected child at school.

## Talking with teenagers

Educating adolescents about sex has always been difficult for many parents. Adding HIV and AIDS to the mix makes it even tougher and even more important. Sex and drugs aren't just dangerous now, they can be deadly. Kids as young as twelve are experimenting with both. Without information about safe sex and clean needles, these children are at great risk for HIV infection. It only takes one mistake to destroy a young person's future.

Adolescence is a time to begin wrestling with grown-up questions. It is also a time when the world seems very open, when the possibilities of life seem endless. Most adolescents have the sense that they are immortal, that nothing can stop them. This attitude is one of the biggest barriers you face in teaching your children about AIDS.

Since teenagers feel like they will live forever, they assume that AIDS can't happen to them, that they are magically immune. Be sure to address this attitude with your kids, and try to help them understand that AIDS does not recognize the charms of youth. It can—and does—happen to anyone.

## *Get the facts*

Before you talk to your teenager about HIV and AIDS, you should make sure you have the facts. Chapters One and Two gave you the basic facts about HIV and how it spreads, as well as resources for finding out more. The most important message to get across to your teen is that AIDS can happen to them. These are the messages your children must get:

* Waiting to become sexually active is the best way to protect yourself.
* If you have sex, use a condom every time.
* Don't shoot up.
* If you do shoot up, use a clean needle. Don't share dirty needles.
* It's okay to say no to sex.
* It's okay to insist on using a condom. It might save your life.
* If you are drunk or high, it's much harder to be safe.

## *Plan your strategy*

Talking with teens is often much more difficult than talking with younger children. Not only is there a greater emphasis on topics like sex and drugs, there is also likely to be more resistance from teens. Adolescence is a time of rebellion and mistrust of adults, particularly parents. This can make your job much tougher.

As you plan your approach, it often helps to get advice from friends and family members or even from a counselor or minister. Your child's school may have resources available as well, including teachers, guidance counselors, or school nurses. These professionals can offer great advice on the best way to talk with your teenager about AIDS, but only you can decide which approach is most comfortable for you.

Remember, although you may want to plan your approach, be sure not to sound canned when you bring the subject up with your children. Start a dialogue with them that is warm and comfortable, one in which they can ask questions and share their feelings. Because the issues around talking with teens about HIV and AIDS are complex, you need more than a standard set of questions and answers about HIV and AIDS. As a parent, you must be willing to respond to anything your adolescent might bring up. Having the facts is vital, but you should spend some time thinking about the emotional and social issues involved with AIDS and how you want to represent them, as well as your own views, to your teenager.

### Bring it up now

Some parents make the mistake of waiting for their teenager to bring up the subject of AIDS. Don't wait! Your child might never bring it up. He or she might feel shy or embarrassed or may fear that you will be angry. The best time to talk to your child is now and the best way to bring up the subject is in a warm and loving manner.

### Ask what they know

When you do talk, it is good to get an idea of how much your children know already. You can help to correct any incorrect information they may have, and they just might teach you something. When asking adolescents about what they know, be sure to use open-ended questions. For example, do not ask whether they know everything they need to know about HIV and AIDS. This closes off the discussion and does not allow you to assess the amount of their knowledge or the accuracy of it. Instead, ask what they know and how they feel.

### Share facts and feelings

As you discuss the facts about HIV transmission with your teen, it's good to acknowledge that these are not the easiest topics to discuss. You may both feel a little embar-

66

rassed—and that's all right. Sharing these feelings of embarrassment or discomfort with each other can help to prompt other types of emotional sharing and thus strengthen the relationship you have with your teen.

This is also a good time for you to talk about your feelings about sex and drugs. If you feel strongly about the need to wait for sex or about any other related issues, let your children know that. Just make sure you give them all the facts. It is important that you acknowledge that they—not you—will be making choices for their lives, but that you want them to make educated choices.

### Set the tone

Make sure you set the right tone for your discussion about HIV and AIDS. Some tips for setting the tone are:

* Treat your son or daughter like a partner—don't talk down.
* Be straightforward and open about the facts.
* Don't use euphemisms—call a condom a condom.
* Use humor—it helps break the ice and relaxes you both.
* Don't preach—don't lay down the law unless you want it broken.
* Create a safe space—make it all right to say anything.

## Use teachable moments

A discussion about HIV and AIDS doesn't need to be a formal affair that takes place at a special time or location. The subject can come up naturally, perhaps as a result of a story on the news, a movie plot, an offhand comment, or anything else. Times like these, in which the issue comes up naturally and you have an opening for good discussion, are known as teachable moments. They are a real opportunity for learning and sharing.

## Show you care

Being a good listener will help you build a trusting relationship with young people, and will make them more comfortable coming to you with problems and concerns, whether HIV-related or not.

## Remember self-esteem

Adolescence is a time of self-discovery. Changing from a child to an adult can be turbulent and challenging. Deciding who you are can lead to many crises. Questions like, Am I attractive? and Will I fit in? are very important in the life of a teenager. These questions take on great significance when asked in the context of safer sex. Imagine your teen's questions in light of a sexual experience: Will he think I'm uncool if I insist on a condom? and Will this

wreck the mood? Will I seem unromantic or unpassion-
ate? Will I be rejected? Merely knowing how to put on a
condom is not enough. Your teens also need to ensure
that they use a condom every time they have sex. Teens
who have high self-esteem, who feel their own self-worth,
are more likely to want to protect themselves than teens
who do not.

Just as the teen years are a time of confusion about
and movement toward a sense of self, they are also a time
for explorations of sexuality. Young people who are ques-
tioning whether they are straight or gay often have many
self-esteem issues.

It is estimated that one-third of all teen suicides are
related to sexuality issues and crises. Coming out is a difficult task, even in the best of circumstances, and coming
out to themselves is most difficult for lesbian and gay
teens. Because of the prejudice and stigma associated with
being gay or lesbian in our society, these teens must hide
their feelings, their questions and confusions, even their
romantic relationships and attractions. As a parent, it is
vital that you be aware of this potential and that you offer
support and encouragement for your teen, regardless of
orientation. Your son or daughter's life may well depend
on it.

*Acknowledge—and accept—your limitations*

So, you've followed all these steps. You've thought about what you need to say about HIV and AIDS and how best to say it. You've worked up your courage and steeled your nerves, and . . . you just can't do it. Or, you did it. You brought the topic up, but it just didn't go over well at all. Your teenage son or daughter didn't want to hear it, at least not from you. What should a parent do?

It's important to remember that teens usually aren't responsive to authority, particularly that of Mom and Dad. The teen years are about breaking free and becoming independent—probably more independent than you would like. This is a fact of adolescence, just like hormones, mood swings, and pimples. But as a parent, you want to be sure that your child gets the message about HIV and AIDS, even though you may not be the best person to deliver it.

Give your adolescent the opportunity to learn from other educational forums. There are many excellent groups and resources trying to educate teens about AIDS. Supporting their efforts and encouraging your child to use them is a positive and effective step for you to take. You can be actively involved in your child's AIDS education without being the one to teach them how to put on a condom. Here are some ways to get involved:

✳ SUPPORT PEER EDUCATION. Peer education efforts, or kids teaching kids, are tremendously effective. Support the work of your local health department, Red Cross or Planned Parenthood chapter, or other AIDS service organization involved in teen peer education.

✳ WORK WITH THE SCHOOL SYSTEM. Public schools have some sort of state-mandated HIV education curriculum. Find out what it is and how you can support the schools in teaching it. If the instruction offered is not enough or you do not think it is sound, write or call the school board and suggest ways to strengthen it.

✳ WORK WITH OTHER PARENTS. Use your role as a Parent-Teacher Association (PTA) member or team booster to connect with other parents. Make sure they know the facts and understand the importance of HIV and AIDS education for teens. Help raise their awareness of the issue and encourage their compassion.

Even though you may not be the one teaching your children about AIDS, you are still involved in their education. Be sure to let them know that you care, that you want to play a role, and that you realize the best role for you is one behind the scenes. Make sure your child knows that you are available.

# LEARNING MORE ABOUT TALKING WITH YOUR CHILDREN ABOUT HIV AND AIDS

### Books for parents

*AIDS-Proofing Your Kids: A Step-by-Step Guide* by LOREN E. ACKER, BRAM C. GOLDWATER, and WILLIAM H. DYSON (Beyond Words, 1992)

*Children and the AIDS Virus: A Book for Children, Parents, and Teachers* by ROSMARIE HAUSHERR (Houghton Mifflin, 1989)

*Does AIDS Hurt?* by MARCIA QUACKENBUSH (ETR Associates, 1988)

*How to Talk to Your Kids About Really Important Things: Specific Questions, Answers and Useful Things to Say* by CHARLES E. SCHAEFER AND THERESA DeGERONIMO (Jossey-Bass, 1993)

*Parents' Guide to Risky Times* by BETH WINSHIP (Workman, 1990)

*Talking with Your Child About a Troubled World* by LYNNE S. DUMAS (Fawcett, 1992)

For a free booklet on talking to your children about AIDS, send a self-addressed, stamped envelope to:

DEPARTMENT OF HEALTH EDUCATION
SIECUS / New York University, Dept. BHG
32 Washington Place
New York, NY 10003

### Books for children

*AIDS and Drugs* by NICHOLAS BEVAN (F. Watts, 1988)

*AIDS: How It Works in the Body* by LORNA GREENBERG (F. Watts, 1992)

*AIDS Questions and Answers for Kids* by LINDA SCHWARTZ (Learning Works, revised edition, 1993)

*AIDS: You Can't Catch It Holding Hands* by NIKI DE SAINT PHALLE (Lapis Press, 1987)

*Alex, the Kid with AIDS* by LINDA WALVOORD GIRARD (A. Whitman, 1991)

*Come Sit by Me* by MARGARET MERRIFIELD (Woman's Press, 1990)

*Losing Uncle Tim* by MARY KATE JORDAN (A. Whitman, 1989)

*Ryan White, My Own Story* by RYAN WHITE and ANN MARIE CUNNINGHAM (Dial Books, 1991)

*When Someone Dies* by SHARON GREENLEE (Peachtree, 1992)

### Resources for adolescents

*AIDS: Trading Fears for Facts* by KAREN HEIN and THERESA FOY DIGERONIMO (Consumer Reports Books, 1993)

*100 Questions and Answers About AIDS: What You Need to Know Now* by MICHAEL THOMAS FORD (Beech Tree Press, 1994)

*Risky Times* by JEANNE BLAKE (Workman, 1990)

*Time Out: The Truth About HIV, AIDS, and You* with MAGIC JOHNSON and ARSENIO HALL (videotape)

*What You Can Do to Avoid AIDS* by EARVIN "MAGIC" JOHNSON (Times Books, 1992)

# How Should I Act Around People with AIDS?

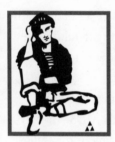

We get nervous. We avoid the subject. We look away. We don't want to know. We may not like to admit this to ourselves, but we don't really like to talk about AIDS, and worse still, we don't know how to act around people with AIDS. We'd rather avoid them.

AIDS forces us to confront parts of life we are uncomfortable with, like sexuality, sickness, and death. People with AIDS know all of this. They know that their friends avoid certain subjects with them. They notice that people stop touching them. They hear us talk about "innocent victims of AIDS" and wonder if they are among the guilty. They feel themselves gradually being pushed outside, not called, left alone, cast off by society.

It's normal to have some fear or troubling thoughts and uncertainties about what to do or say. You shouldn't be ashamed. Everyone is unsure of how to act in new situations. If you haven't known anyone with a fatal disease before, you're probably not going to know what to do when you first meet someone who does.

In the first two chapters we learned that you can't catch HIV just by being near people with AIDS—not by touching them, hugging them, or doing any of the things friends normally do together. In this chapter, we will learn about important considerations to make when getting to know people who are living with AIDS.

While we should be aware of some basic health issues and special sensitivities people with AIDS might have, there is no need to learn any special new kind of behavior to use with them. We only need to treat them with the same respect and humanity with which, ideally, we treat everyone. There are, however, a few wrong assumptions many of us make about what to say or do around people with AIDS that can lead to thoughtless and mistaken characterizations and prejudgment. What then, is the best way to reach out to people living with AIDS? The following suggestions should help.

## *Get to know people living with AIDS*

Knowing people who are living with HIV helps to humanize the disease and allows you to see beyond the staggering headlines and statistics. AIDS isn't really about numbers and risk groups—it's about people, about friends and family, co-workers and caregivers.

Most of us are afraid or unsure of ourselves in unfamiliar situations. We also may feel uncomfortable around, or have wrong ideas about, people we don't know. AIDS is a scary disease. People who have AIDS may seem scary as well. The obvious way to solve this problem is to get to know some people living with AIDS.

It's important to remember the difference between being HIV positive and having AIDS. People who are HIV positive may be healthy; they often look just like everyone else. You probably already know people who are HIV positive, and you just are not aware of it. Unless people tell you their HIV status, you can't tell who has been infected. You can meet people with HIV anywhere—on the job, at a baseball game, at the grocery store—anywhere you meet people.

Those who have been diagnosed with AIDS, however, are beginning to feel—and show—the effects of a weakened immune system. As the disease progresses, they may

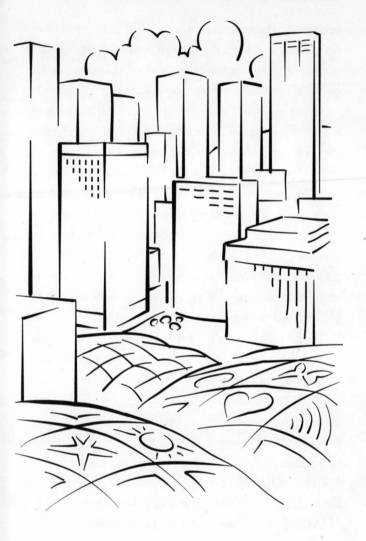

need more assistance and support. These are probably the people you will meet if you begin volunteering for AIDS service organizations, whether you are delivering meals, providing practical support, or visiting the AIDS ward.

There are many ways to learn about AIDS and how it affects the lives of those who live with it. A good first step is to read books, watch documentaries, or even read plays by or about people with AIDS. Your local library probably has a number of the excellent books listed in the back of this chapter. Many video stores rent films like *Philadelphia* or *Longtime Companion* and documentaries such as *Common Threads: Stories from the Quilt,* a film about the AIDS Memorial Quilt. These works contain many inspiring and moving stories about the lives of people with AIDS, their caregivers, and families.

Many people have their first exposure to the people behind the statistics at a display of the AIDS Memorial Quilt. The quilt is a giant, ever-growing fabric memorial made up of thousands of three-by-six-foot panels, each remembering the life of a person lost to AIDS. Each panel, created by family, friends, and lovers, tells the story of a life and helps to build awareness and compassion. Portions of the quilt are displayed in communities all over the country. For information about the quilt, contact The NAMES Project Foundation at 415/882-5500.

As the disease takes hold in more communities across the country and around the world, it becomes more and more likely that you will know someone who is affected by AIDS—a friend, a co-worker, even a family member. If AIDS has not yet touched your life so personally, you may want to become acquainted with people who are living with AIDS. Once you have an understanding of AIDS as a force in the lives of individuals and not just as a faraway and terrifying plague, you may feel ready to become involved in the fight against the disease.

One of the best and most helpful ways to get to know a person with AIDS is to volunteer for an AIDS service organization in your community. There are many ways to make a difference. For instance, you can deliver meals to people with AIDS, work at a drop-in center, or help to provide practical or emotional support to people who are living with the disease.

Elly, a woman in Washington, D.C., wanted to experience directly what she had been reading about in the papers, so she volunteered through a church group to clean house for people with AIDS. Through this program she met Lillian, a young woman with AIDS. Elly says:

*"When I decided to help I had a lot of built-in expectations. I thought I'd meet people that were really different. I never imagined I'd meet a woman who was dealing*

80

*with the disease, a woman who reminds me of myself. Meeting Lillian has really opened my eyes and helped me to see that AIDS can happen to anyone."*

Chapter Five discusses volunteering at AIDS service organizations and describes the types of volunteer services that are needed.

## Don't misspeak about AIDS

Language and how we use it is very important. It reveals a lot about what we think and how we feel. When talking about AIDS, there are a number of disrespectful and dehumanizing words we may use unintentionally.

### There are no "AIDS victims"

One of the most important changes we should make is to stop using the term victim to refer to people who are living with AIDS. By calling someone an AIDS victim we are saying that he or she is powerless in the face of this disease and should have no hope. We should instead use our words to emphasize the strength and the hope of those fighting AIDS.

### There are no "innocent victims"

Early in the epidemic—and even today, unfortunately—it was common for people to talk about the "innocent vic-

tims" of AIDS who caught the disease "through no fault
of their own." This implied that anyone who caught the
disease because of doing something unsafe was some sort
of guilty perpetrator of AIDS who deserved to suffer a
terrible death. This sort of judgment, which casts some as
innocent and lays blame on others, serves only to increase
the stigma attached to this awful disease. No one with
AIDS deserves to have it. No one deserves to suffer.

### There are just people with AIDS

What you call someone is important. A name signifies
more than just the words used, it suggests how the individual being referred to is seen by the group. People are
often confused about what to call a person living with
AIDS. If the term victim is out, what can you say? Most
say, simply, "person with AIDS," which is often shortened
to "PWA." Others even make it "PLWA" or "person living with AIDS." These phrases and acronyms help to
maintain the humanity of the person involved, and they
avoid reducing anyone to a diagnosis or condition.

### Do not ask how a person caught HIV

It's tactless to ask how a person got AIDS. It implies
that some of the ways of contracting the virus are all right
and others are not. It's like asking someone if they are an

innocent victim or if they deserved it. This question serves no real purpose and gets in the way of getting to know a person living with AIDS.

## Be yourself: behave normally toward people with AIDS

Now that we know AIDS can't be spread by casual contact, how do we relax enough to be casual with a person who has AIDS? Many people become very nervous about this. Worrying that they might offend or upset, they find it hard to relax and behave naturally. People with AIDS will be much more upset by distance and restraint than by anything you might say. Treat people with AIDS with respect and awareness, not with velvet gloves.

### Don't be afraid to touch

Humans crave touch. Being touched is comforting; it's one of the ways we know that we are liked and trusted by others. Without touch, there is less reinforcement, less comfort, less love. Without touch, there is a sense of isolation, of being alone. Because so many people are afraid of touching them, people with AIDS miss out on this ordinary physical contact. Hugging and shaking hands are completely safe and can make a huge difference in the life of someone with AIDS.

### *Don't be afraid of saying the wrong thing*

Although it is important to learn about respectful language and other sensitivities, these issues should not stop people from making contact. The main challenge is to not behave differently toward people with AIDS. When you make a genuine attempt to know someone, your friendly intention makes more of an impact than a few wrong words ever could.

### *Understand that anyone can have AIDS*

AIDS crosses all lines of gender, race, class, and sexuality. It is not simply a gay disease. While it is true that gay men were among the first and hardest hit, AIDS has spread far beyond this community. Gays and lesbians responded very publicly and heroically to the epidemic; they began many of the AIDS services and resources currently available. While the gay and lesbian response has been inspiring, the public has been less receptive to AIDS information because it perceives AIDS as a gay disease. This attitude not only stigmatizes those living with AIDS, it leads to unnecessary risk-taking, poor choices, and the spread of fear and hatred in our society.

If you see AIDS as a disease that only touches other people's lives, you probably won't take the precautions

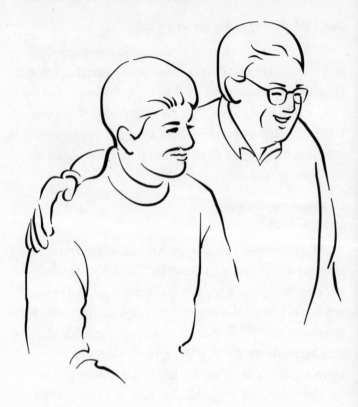

that could save your own life. You may also think of those who are infected with HIV or living with AIDS as different or as deserving of their fate. The AIDS epidemic provides an opportunity to accept others and to practice compassion.

If you know someone who has AIDS—if not a friend, perhaps a friend of a friend, a friend's family member, and so on—you may wonder if your relationship with that person will change. Remember, a person's personality doesn't change when disease strikes. They still have the same likes, dislikes, and sense of humor. Also, like anyone who is facing a terminal illness, a person with AIDS wants and deserves to be treated with respect, dignity and, most importantly, without pity. It's important to keep this in mind when relating to people with AIDS.

Pity is an emotion that may seem loving or kind to the one who feels it, but which feels very different to the

"When I first met my caregiver, Margaret, she was very sweet, although a little nervous around me. I think I was her first gay acquaintance, as well as her first experience with AIDS. She seemed afraid of asking the wrong thing or saying something to offend me. After a few times together, though, she loosened up and began asking questions about my life and experiences. Now she's really open and we can talk about anything." —JOHN, A PERSON LIVING WITH AIDS

person on the receiving end. It is kinder to ask "May I help you?" than to say "Do you need help with that?" No one wants to feel patronized or condescended to; no one likes feeling powerless or like a burden.

## Be aware of special health needs

There are many things we take for granted in our daily lives, such as the ability of our immune system to fight off ever-present germs, or being able to move comfortably in many environments. But for someone with an immune weakness, the environment presents many challenges and hazards. People with AIDS have special health needs that force them to worry daily about things most of us never even think about. There are a number of things we can do to make life easier—and more healthy—for people with AIDS, both in our homes and offices.

❋ DON'T GO TO WORK SICK. When you go to work sick, you not only run yourself down and increase your own recovery time, you may also give what you have to co-workers. Since people with AIDS have a tough time fighting off infections, keeping your cold and flu bugs at home helps everyone stay healthier.

❋ PROVIDE A HEALTHY SPACE. A healthy environment is good for everyone and can help reduce the risk of spreading common colds, flus, and more serious infections among all people, including people with AIDS or HIV. Make sure there is adequate ventilation at home and in the workplace, and keep things clean, particularly in kitchens and bathrooms. Bacterial and fungal infections that are airborne or spread on surfaces can be very damaging to people with weakened immune systems. Make sure that air-conditioning filters are cleaned regularly and that thermostats are not set too low.

> "HIV takes such a toll on the immune system that folks who live with it need to pay special attention to things like germs and bacteria that most of us wouldn't be bothered by."
> —CAROL, A VIRAL CLINIC NURSE

✳ AVOID STRONG SCENTS IN PERSONAL CARE AND HOUSEHOLD PRODUCTS. Strong scents can be overpowering to someone with a weakened immune system. Do not, for example, overdo the cologne or the air freshener.

✳ DON'T SERVE RISKY FOODS. Avoid undercooked, unwashed, or potentially spoiled foods, since people with AIDS are more sensitive to harmful bacteria than healthy people are. Good foods for people with compromised immune systems are basically the same foods that are healthy for the rest of us, including lots of fruits, vegetables, and whole grains. Be sure to wash foods that may have been chemically treated. Some foods to avoid are: Unpasteurized milk, dairy products, or soft, ripened cheeses (like Camembert); raw fish, meats, and eggs (sushi, oysters, eggnogs); undercooked meats; and aged foods, such as cheeses, sausage, or moldy items.

✳ HAVE NONCAFFEINATED BEVERAGES AVAILABLE. While caffeinated beverages seem to be what makes the world go 'round, they can be harmful to the health of people with AIDS. Be sure to have noncaffeinated options, such as herbal teas, available.

✳ KEEP PET WASTE OUT OF THE WAY. Although animals can be a tremendous source of love and joy for people living with AIDS, handling their waste products can be dangerous—even deadly. Toxoplasmosis, a serious fungal infection that leads to seizures, coma, and death, is spread most commonly through cleaning out kitty litter. Psittacosis is an infectious disease-causing organism that is spread through bird feces.

# Learning More About People Living with AIDS

### Books about the experience of AIDS

*Anonymity: The Secret Life of an American Family* by Susan Bergman (Farrar, Straus & Giroux, 1994)

*Borrowed Time: An AIDS Memoir* by Paul Monette (Avon Books, 1988)

*In the Absence of Angels* by Elisabeth Glaser and Laura Palmer (Berkley, 1992)

*Positive Women: Voices of Women Living with AIDS* edited by Andrea Rudd and Darien Taylor (Second Story Press, 1992)

*A Promise to Remember: The NAMES Project Book of Letters* edited by Joe Brown (Avon, 1992)

*The Quilt: Stories from The NAMES Project* by Cindy Ruskin (Pocket Books, 1988)

*A Rock and a Hard Place: One Boy's Triumphant Story* by Anthony Godby Johnson (Crown, 1993)

*Ryan White: My Own Story* by Ryan White and Ann Marie Cunningham (Dial Books, 1991)

*The Screaming Room: A Mother's Journal of her Son's Struggle with AIDS* by Barbara Peabody (Avon, 1986)

*Seasons of Grief and Grace: A Sister's Story of AIDS* by Susan Ford Wiltshire (Vanderbilt, 1994)

*Sleep with the Angels: A Mother Challenges AIDS* by Mary Fisher (Moyer Bell, 1994)

*Someone Was Here: Profiles in the AIDS Epidemic* by GEORGE WHITMORE (NAL Books, 1988)

*Surviving AIDS* by MICHAEL CALLEN (Harper Perennial, 1990)

*Thanksgiving: An AIDS Journal* by ELIZABETH COX (HarperCollins, 1990)

**Videotapes about the experience of AIDS**

*Common Threads: Stories from the Quilt*
*Philadelphia*
*Longtime Companion*
*The Los Altos Story*

# Helping People Living with AIDS

 Like anyone living with a
serious illness, people
with AIDS need help.
They need help in caring
for their health, taking
their medicine, preparing their food,
and going to the doctor. They need
help maintaining the quality of their
lives, the beauty of their surroundings,
and the order of their homes.

As you've already read several times in this book, maintaining a positive attitude is crucial to living with AIDS. Like everyone else, people with AIDS feel better if they get a lot of support and if the quality of their life does not unnecessarily deteriorate.

Helping people with AIDS is one of the best ways to feel actively and directly involved in the fight against AIDS. No matter who you are and what you can do, you can help people who are living with AIDS. You can provide emotional support through counseling and activity programs or practical support by delivering meals and running errands. You can get involved helping people you know directly or through an AIDS service organization. Most service organizations rely heavily on volunteers to help with all the services they provide.

This chapter will discuss ways of using your skills and interests to make a difference in the lives of people with AIDS.

## *Be a "buddy"*

— — — — — — — — — — —

Helping people with AIDS is rewarding, but it can also be very challenging. Special training in being an AIDS caregiver, often called "buddy training," is offered by various organizations, such as your state AIDS Project. (See the back of the book for a listing of state AIDS telephone numbers.) This type of training can give you the skills and the knowledge you need to support a person with AIDS effectively. Buddy training also gives you an idea of what to expect and helps you prepare to meet the challenges of AIDS before you actually have to face them. During this training, you will learn the basic medical facts about the disease and how it spreads. This knowledge will not only give you an idea of what to expect but will help you understand what your buddy is dealing with physically as well.

### Communication skills

One of the most important aspects of caregiver training is learning—and refining—communication skills. People can become better listeners; they can become more able to define and clarify feelings, and, as a result, be better able to cope with potentially difficult communication issues. Training also places a strong emphasis on the

94 concept of confidentiality. The privacy of people with AIDS should be protected. Maintaining confidentiality is part of being involved in an effective helping relationship.

### Death and dying

Since AIDS is not currently a curable condition, people with AIDS and their caregivers need to face the realities of loss and grief. As you learn about providing support for people with AIDS, you will have to examine your feelings about death and dying. In preparing to join the fight against AIDS, you will need to think about how it will feel to be involved with a terminally ill person and how you will deal with the loss of the person you have worked with.

### Stress management

Your training course will also teach effective ways of managing the stress you and the person you are caring for will feel. Many techniques can help you work through difficult situations and maintain the positive attitude that is vital to everyone's health during a difficult time.

### *Crisis management*

Crisis management skills, taught in many training programs, can help you cope with many immediate crises, such as medical emergencies, emotional outbursts, or financial difficulties. Crisis training also shows you how to help cope with common crises in the life of a person with AIDS, such as an allergic reaction to medications or treatments, the onset of new symptoms, or the death of a loved one.

96 *Provide emotional support*

People living with AIDS are often afraid of being and dying alone. They feel great sadness and grief, perhaps guilt, or even shame and anger. They need emotional support as they face the changes in their lives. There are a variety of ways to provide emotional support to people with AIDS.

### Counseling

People with AIDS face complex emotional issues and feelings. They need support in their struggles, as well as information and assistance in dealing with the many frustrating and frightening aspects of life with AIDS. A caregiver trained to give emotional support can be an invaluable member of a sick person's total support network. Even those without special training may be called upon to provide a listening ear to a friend with AIDS. People with AIDS face many serious emotional challenges, such as:

❋ DISTRESSING FEELINGS AND LOW SELF-ESTEEM: There are many anxiety-producing emotions, such as fear, anger, or sorrow that can be involved in living with AIDS. Being sick can lead to a poor body image as well as depression over loss of independence.

❋ FACING LOSSES: Studies show that most people facing death go through the predictable stages of grief identified by Elisabeth Kübler-Ross: denial of the terminal condition, anger and resentment, bargaining with God or doctors for more time, depression, and finally, acceptance. In addition, many who are living with AIDS now have lost loved ones to the disease. Accepting the loss of friends and lovers, as well as facing up to one's own mortality, is one of the crucial emotional issues faced by people with AIDS. Others include loss of quality of life, loss of independence, loss of faith in their own body, loss of relationships, loss of control over how time is spent, loss of housing or job, and loss of the ability to think due to dementia.

✳ COPING WITH CRISIS PERIODS: People with AIDS may face many crisis periods, for example during initial diagnosis, onset of illnesses, or failure of treatment.

✳ SEARCHING FOR HOPE: Developing a positive and hopeful attitude is both essential and very challenging. Since AIDS is most often a terminal illness, people with AIDS must balance feelings of despair or hopelessness with a sense of hope. They need to feel as though their life is not over, that they can still make choices and have some degree of control over their situation.

✳ FILLING THE NEED FOR SOCIAL SUPPORT: Maintaining contact with friends and loved ones is important. Unfortunately, some people have been rejected by family or loved ones due to the stigma surrounding AIDS, while others have lost most of their friends to the disease, and are left to face AIDS alone.

✻ OBTAINING SUPPORT DURING MEDICAL TREATMENTS: AIDS involves many medical treatments that are often painful or frightening. Support from others during these difficult times is invaluable.

✻ FACING FINANCIAL INSTABILITY: AIDS is a very costly illness. Even those who have good insurance coverage usually end up spending all of their money on treatments and hospitalizations. As the disease progresses, PWA's are often unable to continue working, which can lead to increased financial instability as well. Fear of having no money is a great emotional weight for those facing the disease.

### Activities

Emotional support doesn't necessarily mean long, tearful conversations. Going to movies, athletic events, plays, parades, concerts, and so on can provide a great emotional boost to people with AIDS. Many organizations sponsor group events. Free tickets can often be arranged as well.

### Being there for holidays

Holidays are times when loneliness and isolation can be most upsetting. Spending time with people with AIDS during important holidays can make a big difference in their lives. You can also make the holidays festive by:

* Helping to decorate the HIV/AIDS ward or a local hospice.
* Filling Thanksgiving baskets with holiday goodies like cranberry sauce, pumpkin pie, minipumpkins, and colorful ears of corn.
* Filling Christmas stockings with fun and useful items, such as sample toiletries (unscented), colored pencils, small gourmet treats, candles, and other little tokens.
* Making sure that friends with AIDS are included at Seder, Thanksgiving, and other holiday feasts. (Remember to consider dietary needs when cooking for PWA's.)

### Reading aloud

Some people who have HIV-disease develop a condition called cytomegalovirus, or CMV, which can affect the vision and make reading difficult or impossible. One way to make a difference for people who have lost their sight and can no longer read is by reading books aloud to them. This is a great way to spend time with them and can be very helpful. Books on tape are also an important resource you can provide to people with AIDS.

### Giving telephone support

If you have trouble with mobility and can't get to the house of a person with AIDS or take him or her out, you

**"I'm 81 years old and can't get out of my house, but I call Richard every day, just to check in. We chat about everything— our health, our families, our favorite soap opera."**
**—EMILY, A PHONE BUDDY**

may wish to keep in touch by phone. This is a great way for homebound or elderly people to get involved. A daily check-in call may help to raise a sick person's spirits and ensure that there is no emergency.

### Cuddling babies

Many infants who are born with HIV never know what it is like to be held by their mothers. Perhaps their mothers are too sick to take care of them or are unable to be part of their infant's life due to drug dependence. Touch is the primary way that babies learn to feel love and the psychological benefits of being held regularly can be great for these babies later in life. Many hospitals have programs for volunteer "snugglers." Kay, a grandmother of four who lives 2,000 miles away from her grandchildren volunteers two mornings a week at the neonatal intensive care unit at her local hospital. During her time at the hospital, she holds HIV-infected babies, giving them the love they so desperately need. As for her, the time with these babies gives her the "kid fix" she needs.

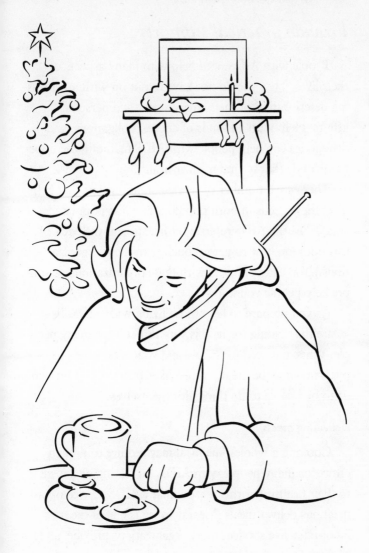

*Provide practical support*

People with AIDS need help with many aspects of their lives. They should not have to put up with a depressing deterioration of their environment and personal affairs. Help with all kinds of chores, obligations, and drudgeries can help people with AIDS maintain the hopeful attitude that is vital to their health.

There are a number of service organizations that help meet these needs in both populous and less-populated areas. (See the AIDS referral information at the back of this book on how to get in touch with these organizations.) You can volunteer with these organizations or simply help people you know.

As you prepare to help those living with AIDS, be aware that asking for help is very difficult for many people. While the need for help—and your willingness to pitch in—may be great, no one likes to feel like a burden or to be unable to do things for themselves.

### Delivering meals

Cooking a wholesome meal may require too much effort for many people with AIDS, but eating well is vital to their health. For this reason, many AIDS service organizations deliver meals. Meal delivery is one of the most labor-intensive services most organizations provide, and

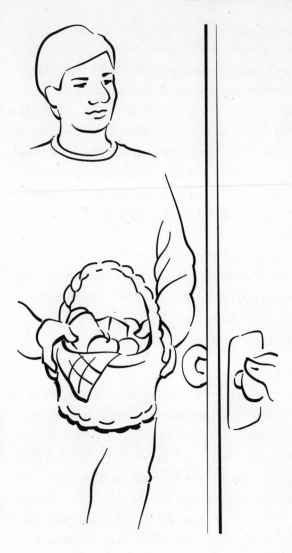

they always need help, especially from people with cars. If there isn't a meal delivery service near you, you can cook and deliver meals yourself or enlist a few friends. Many meal delivery services began in a church basement or in someone's kitchen. If you prepare meals yourself, be aware of special dietary needs that people with AIDS might have. For instance, spicy foods can be difficult for people with AIDS to eat, particularly if they have sores in the mouth. Before you begin preparing meals, you should consult with your local AIDS office for food and nutrition guidelines.

Another important consideration is socialization. Often, meals are easier to eat if they are shared with others. Perhaps you could stay for the meal rather than just dropping it off. Also, if people help in planning their own meals, they may be more interested in eating.

### Caring for pets

Having animal companionship is an important part of many people's lives. Unconditional love from a beloved pet is a great source of comfort. When a person faces a life-threatening disease such as AIDS, this love can play an even more important role because it helps to reduce stress and give support in a way no human can. Since people with AIDS are susceptible to several serious diseases that are spread by cat or bird feces, taking care of the litterbox or cleaning out the birdcage or fish tank is a great way to help. If you are an animal lover and don't mind a little odor, you can make a tremendous difference in the life of a person with AIDS.

Another way to help with pet care is by walking people's dogs when they are unable to do so because of illness.

### Working in the house and garden

A clean and beautiful house or garden can help to cheer up people with AIDS. No one who cares about their home likes to watch it deteriorate around them as their health fails. Some types of cleaning and yard work can also expose people with AIDS to dangerous germs. Any cleaning or beautifying you can do in the home of someone living with AIDS will be greatly appreciated.

Jack, who began getting sick at the same time as his lover, Don, had a lovely garden and many exotic house plants. As he and Don got sicker, they became less and less able to take care of their plants and garden. When Susan, a fellow plant lover and longtime admirer of their garden, heard of their plight, she volunteered to come over frequently to water plants and help with garden maintenance. She also enlisted the help of her two teenagers to mow the lawn and do the weeding. Susan says:

*"I always admired Jack and Don's garden, and when they began to get sick, I knew that helping to keep their*

*garden up was the best possible way to help them out. I also found that, in doing the work as a family, I was able to have some really open and honest discussions about HIV and AIDS with my boys, who are 14 and 17."*

### Running errands

Buying groceries, sending packages, getting things repaired, doing laundry—everyone has a hard time keeping up with these necessary errands. People with AIDS have no fewer errands than others do. In fact they often have more, such as filling prescriptions or dropping off insurance forms. If you're heading downtown to do errands for yourself, ask a person with AIDS if you can bring something back or make a needed stop along the way.

### Driving

For people with AIDS who must rely on public transportation, getting to a medical appointment or picking up a prescription can mean exhausting hours on the bus. Taking people to the doctor, to the pharmacy or even to the supermarket is a great way to help. Remember, if a PWA walks unsteadily, be sure to offer your arm for security and support.

*Paying bills, filling out forms, and other administrative work*

People with AIDS often must do even more paper-work than the rest of us. They must deal with their insurance companies, lawyers, government agencies, and other service providers, along with the ordinary mountain of bills—bills for rent, taxes, utilities, and so on. Many people with AIDS are on medical disability and must cope with a multitude of forms and legal documents. Anyone with administrative skills can be an enormous help.

### Caring for children of people with AIDS

When parents get sick, children don't stop needing care and attention. Children of people with AIDS face a great loss. Getting close to other caregivers can help them prepare for this loss and allow their parents important time for rest.

### Giving coupon books

One way to make it easier for people to ask you to do things for them is to make a little gift book and include coupons for doing dishes, going to the grocery store, driving to appointments, picking up dry cleaning, changing the cat litter, walking the dog, and other helpful tasks. That way, instead of asking for another favor, a person can just cash in a coupon.

108 *Use your skills*

- - - - - - - - - -

Any skill you possess can be useful to a person with AIDS. Whether you are a lawyer, a masseuse, a building contractor, a desktop publisher, or a really good cook, any special talent you have can help someone with AIDS or an organization that provides AIDS services in your area.

Some AIDS service organizations keep listings of volunteers willing to provide free skilled services to people with AIDS. Even when there is no formal arrangement, if you just let people know about services you can provide, the word gets around.

Some examples of people who make a unique contribution based on their special talents are:

✳ VJ, a caterer in the Midwest, is known as the "Muffin Lady." Every Thursday morning, she bakes some of her famous nutritious muffins and delivers them to friends with AIDS in her community.

✳ Tom is an accountant at a large hospital. In the evening, he volunteers at a local AIDS organization helping people with AIDS keep track of their finances and make sense of insurance forms.

✳ Larry directs a youth choir. After years of performing for elderly people in nursing homes, his choir has branched out. Now they perform at AIDS wards and local hospices. Often the children will stay on after the performance and help out on the unit, playing games, helping with mealtimes, and just hanging out.

✳ Emily makes terrific soups. When she makes a big potful, she freezes some in Ziploc bags and gives the bags to a local meal delivery service. These bags can be thawed out and microwaved with little difficulty; they provide a good home-cooked meal for a person dealing with AIDS.

✳ Julie works at a flower shop. Every week she delivers a few colorful flowers to friends with AIDS to brighten their apartments and their days.

110 *Avoid burnout*

When giving care to a person with AIDS, whether you do it every day or just once in a while, it's important to work at a sustainable level. The people who do the most in the long run are those who understand their own needs and work at a level that will not damage their health and well-being. Those who work too hard and martyr themselves to the cause often become casualties in the AIDS war.

AIDS caregivers are faced with unprecedented challenges. In caring for those who live with—and die from—this stigmatized and complex disease, a caregiver must deal with incredible uncertainty and constant change. The health of an ill person can change rapidly, which can lead to feelings of inadequacy for the caregiver. Often, there is nothing to be done, and this sense of impotence can be draining. Over time, these feelings can build up for the caregiver and lead to emotional exhaustion or burnout.

AIDS is also an infectious disease, and while casual contact is completely safe, there may be times when you are giving care to a PWA and bodily fluids are present, which means precautions must be taken. This can lead to natural fears about protecting oneself, fears that must be balanced with the desire to help.

Caregiving is a tough job. It will change your life. It's important not to let it take over your life, however. Some of the biggest considerations to make when you are involved in AIDS work and volunteering are to:

✳ Take time for yourself. You'll come back refreshed, renewed, and more able to make a difference.

✳ Live one day at a time. The outcome of a relationship with a PWA will probably include grief and loss. Make sure you get as much out of each day as possible.

✳ Recognize your limits. Don't try to be a superman or wonder woman.

✳ Seek support from others. Get help any way you can, whether through support groups, counseling, caregiver courses or seminars, friends, or written or taped resources such as those listed at the back of this chapter.

# LEARNING MORE ABOUT HOW TO HELP PEOPLE LIVING WITH AIDS

### Resources on being a caregiver

*The AIDS Caregiver's Handbook* edited by TED EIDSON (St. Martin's Press, 1988)

*AIDS Caregiving: Lessons for the Second Decade* (audiotapes) CHARLES GARFIELD and CINDY SPRING (Jossey-Bass, 1993)

*The Caregiver's Journey: When You Love Someone with AIDS* by MEL POHL, DENISTON KAY and DOUG TOFT (Hazelden, 1990)

*Caring for a Loved One with AIDS: The Experiences of Families, Lovers, and Friends* by MARIE ANNETTE BROWN and GAIL M. POWELL-COPE (University of Washington Press, 1992)

*I Don't Know What to Say: How to Help and Support Someone Who Is Dying* by ROBERT BUCKMAN (Vintage, 1988)

*The Journey Through AIDS: A Guide for Loved Ones and Caregivers* by DEBRA JARVIS (Lion, 1992)

*Take These Broken Wings and Learn to Fly: The Support Book for Patients, Family, and Friends Living with AIDS* by STEVEN D. DIETZ and M. JAMES PARKER HICKS (Harbinger House, 1992)

*When Someone You Know Has AIDS: A Practical Guide* by LEONARD J. MARTELL, FRAN D. PELTZ, WILLIAM MESSINA, and STEVE PETROW (Crown, 1993)

### Books about support groups

*Support Groups: The Human Face of the HIV/AIDS Epidemic* by GAIL BAROUH (LIAAC, 1992)

# Raising Awareness in Your Community

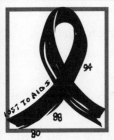

It will not be a heroic individual who defeats AIDS—not a great scientist or a great political leader. When we defeat AIDS it will be as communities working together. By working to raise awareness and taking initiative where we live and work, we can stop AIDS without waiting for a miracle of science.

Still, the challenge is great. AIDS has attacked us where we are weakest—at the boundaries of our society. Divisions of race, class, gender, sexuality, age, culture, and geography have often kept us from responding as we should. While we have ignored what we have thought are other people's problems, while we have failed to reach any consensus, or even to communicate openly about the disease, AIDS has killed thousands who might have been saved if they had been properly educated and cared for. Billions of tax dollars have gone to caring for the sick, when earlier millions spent on education and prevention might have stopped AIDS before it spread.

Reaching the awareness and consensus that could lead to a compassionate and coordinated response is perhaps the greatest challenge of the epidemic. When we succeed, we will have taken a great step forward. That's why it's crucial that we work in our communities to promote AIDS awareness and compassion. Most people do respond generously if they are educated. Every effort to raise consciousness saves lives.

When we work in our communities, it's important that we respect local values and traditions. What works in the inner cities may not work in suburbs or rural areas. Always work in the community in ways that will reach people, not irritate or anger them. The sections that follow suggest many ways of approaching different communities.

## *Be an advocate*

- - - - - - - - - -

An advocate doesn't have to be a troublemaker, an agitator, or even an extrovert. An advocate is simply someone who is willing to speak out, and who informs and involves others. If you educate yourself and share your AIDS knowledge with others, you're already an advocate.

Here are some basic ways to advocate for AIDS awareness:

✳ Learn all you can.

✳ Share your knowledge with your friends and family.

✳ Politely speak out when you encounter ignorance, prejudice, and misinformation about AIDS.

✳ Work one-to-one. Some of the most important work is done at this level. This could mean persuading a friend to join in volunteer efforts or talking your boss into starting an AIDS awareness program at work.

✳ Work with groups. You don't have to be a great inspirational speaker. A low-key, informative approach, such as making a simple announcement about available materials or upcoming public events, may be the best way to reach some people.

One of the best places to get basic educational materials is from the CDC. You can get brochures and pamphlets about HIV and AIDS that are suitable for any reader. To contact the CDC National AIDS/HIV Hot Line, call 800/342-2437. This number is answered around the clock and offers resources and assistance with HIV and AIDS information.

For more written HIV and AIDS materials that can be used in AIDS advocacy, contact:

IMPACT AIDS INC.
3692 18th Street
San Francisco, CA 94110
415/861-3397

CENTER FOR HEALTH
INFORMATION
P.O. Box 4636
Foster City, CA 94404
415/345-6669

# Encourage local media to cover AIDS issues

- - - - - - - - - - - -

Most people first learn how AIDS is affecting their community through the local media. Local television and radio stations and newspapers are major sources of AIDS information—and misinformation. As an advocate for AIDS awareness, you should help make sure that the media are covering AIDS both accurately and in depth. Here are some ways to ensure that your local media are being responsive to the needs of the community:

✳ LET THEM KNOW WHAT YOU EXPECT. Write or call local newspapers and radio and television stations to let them know that you appreciate accurate and thorough coverage of AIDS issues.

✳ PAT THEM ON THE BACK. If they publish or broadcast a good story, call to tell them you liked it.

✳ GIVE THEM A PIECE OF YOUR MIND. If they're ignoring the issue or misinforming people, let them know, and tell them you and your neighbors will cancel your subscriptions or watch and listen to other stations.

✳ SPEAK OUT. Write letters to the newspaper editor or tape public service announcements. All television stations are required by law to provide time for such announcements.

Kirsten is a sophomore in college, majoring in broadcasting and film. She and a group of friends made an AIDS awareness video using their community as an example; the video was broadcast over a five-day period during the five and ten o'clock news at a local television station.

"We made the video to help get the word out about AIDS in our town, especially to kids and people who don't think it can happen to them. We interviewed people with AIDS at a local drop-in center, as well as volunteers at the independent testing site and the AIDS ward. We even interviewed my little brother and his friends about what they knew about HIV and condoms. One of my professors knew the station manager at Channel 4 and convinced him to screen the video. He liked it and ran it on the news. The response was really positive."—KIRSTEN, COLLEGE SOPHOMORE

## *Enlist local businesses*

Encourage local businesses to get involved. Merchants can post fliers, help distribute educational materials, or make other contributions. Reward cooperative merchants with your patronage, and encourage your friends and neighbors to do the same.

Form a consumers' group that patronizes businesses that support AIDS causes. Distribute buttons or bumper stickers to your group to show your buying clout. Provide supportive merchants with placards of endorsement from your group.

Encourage merchants to donate a portion of their sales to an AIDS cause, and help promote the merchant's business.

Richard, an AIDS advocate in Chicago, convinced his neighborhood dry cleaner to donate 10 percent of its profits for a month to a local AIDS service organization. With help from Richard's promotional efforts, the dry cleaner actually made more money that month, even after the donation.

"I've been going to this same dry cleaner for years, and I know he values my business. When I suggested that he help out with this promotion, and explained what the cause was all about, he was pretty willing to help out. Since it was done in February, we planned a whole promotion around Valentine's Day and 'having a heart' for people with AIDS." —RICHARD, AIDS ADVOCATE

# Work with your local school and school board

- - - - - - - - - - -

Involving teachers and administrators can make a difference, but to really promote systemwide change in your local schools, you need to work with the school board. Because AIDS is such a controversial issue, it's often difficult for individual educators and school administrators to take the lead.

School boards must confront two main issues: They must (1) ensure that basic information about HIV and AIDS is taught at all levels of schooling, and (2) help create an environment in which HIV-positive staff members and students are treated with compassion.

You may face considerable resistance when approaching some school boards, particularly if you are advocating better sex education or more frequent condom use. Many people still believe that this type of education will encourage students to have sex or use drugs. You should emphasize in a respectful way that AIDS education does not promote or condone sex or drug use and that compassion toward people with AIDS does not present any health risk. Remind them that whether teachers and parents like it or not, teenagers are having sex. Ask them whether they would rather their teens have safe or unsafe sex.

Here are some suggestions to help motivate a school board and ensure an appropriate response:

✳ MEET WITH BOARD MEMBERS PRIVATELY. Arrange private, informal meetings with key members of your local school board and bring along a few friends. You will be more successful in making your opinion known in this setting than at large, impassioned public meetings. If you get board members' support ahead of time, there may not be the need for any public confrontation.

✳ GO TO SCHOOL BOARD MEETINGS. If you do go to public meetings, take a polite group of concerned people along with you to show that you represent a considerable portion of the community. You may want to take some students along to give their viewpoints. Representatives from AIDS organizations can also lend their presence and support to these types of meetings.

✳ LOOK TO OTHER DISTRICTS. Find out what other school districts are doing. If they're doing nothing, approach your district leaders and ask them to assume leadership in the region on these issues. If other districts have good programs, ask for written information and pass this along to your school board. School boards will be more willing to act when they find out there is a clear precedent for such action. Also, they can learn from the experiences of other districts and save themselves a lot of work in forming policies.

For help in working with your school board, contact:

LAMBDA LEGAL DEFENSE AND EDUCATION FUND:
212/995-8585

AMERICAN CIVIL LIBERTIES UNION:
212/944-9800

NATIONAL SCHOOL BOARDS ASSOCIATION:
703/838-6756

NATIONAL EDUCATION ASSOCIATION:
212/833-4000

## *Organize or participate in events*

Certain types of events can focus attention on AIDS in a positive way and bring the community together around the issue. You can participate, or perhaps you can even organize these events.

### Attend or organize healing services and candlelight vigils

Public healing services for those living with AIDS and candlelight vigils to honor those lost to AIDS are deeply moving and inspiring events. They can help bring a community together and motivate it to take action. Bringing forth the names of those with AIDS in this positive way can help remove the stigma surrounding AIDS in some communities.

> "I don't think I really felt how many people we've lost right here in this city—how many sad people there are left alone because AIDS killed their partners. When I went to the vigil and saw all these people holding hands in groups and half of them crying, I really felt it for the first time. I was inspired." —GREG, SAN FRANCISCO

### Host a display of the AIDS Memorial Quilt

The AIDS Memorial Quilt is one of the most poignant, moving, and effective means for raising AIDS awareness. Quilt displays can be very small—a few panels in the

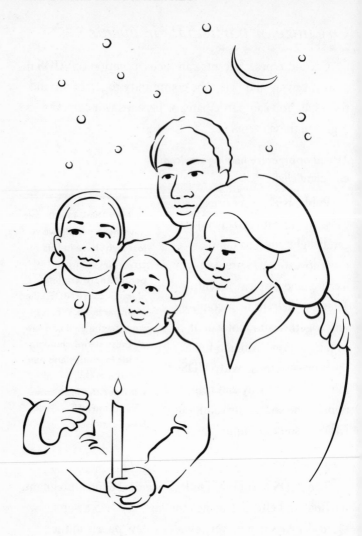

lobby of your workplace—or huge. At the international display of the entire quilt in Washington, D.C., in October 1992, the quilt contained more than twenty thousand panels and blanketed the grounds of the Washington Monument. Bringing the quilt to your community provides an excellent forum for education, for raising public awareness, and remembering local people who have died. In addition, all the money raised during a display of the quilt stays in the community to help fight AIDS.

> "It's amazing how many panels there are from our little town. I can't believe it." —BILL, BOULDER

For information about the quilt and about bringing it to your community, contact The Names Project Foundation at 415/882-5500.

## Host speakers

Invite people with AIDS, people who have lost someone to AIDS, or anyone with valuable knowledge or experience to speak to a group you are a member of. You can even host the event in your own home.

The National Association of People with AIDS (NAPWA) maintains a list of speakers around the country who can speak on many aspects of living with AIDS and caregiving. You may contact them at: 202/898-0414.

126 *Write a newsletter*

Write and distribute a simple newsletter (or write an article for an existing newsletter) containing information about developments in the local AIDS community, needs of service organizations, and so on.

*Launch food and grocery drives*

> "A food drive doesn't have to be a big deal. I just got a big box and put it by the door at my work and put up a sign that said 'Donate grains, canned and dried foods to people with AIDS.'"— LINDA, FRESNO

Have people bring food or other groceries to the office, school, club, bar, or meetings. Donate the food to an AIDS service organization. Be sure to ask the recipients what kind of food or household goods (personal care, housewares, cleaning supplies, and so on) they need most.

*Organize a World AIDS Day event*

World AIDS Day, December 1st, is an international day of remembrance of those lost to AIDS and attention to those living with the disease. Around the world, communities come together for vigils, marches, ceremonies, and many other types of events to acknowledge the tragedy of AIDS. Any of the events discussed already can be planned to coincide with World AIDS Day. Local media may be more attentive to your actions if they coincide with events going on around the world. The American Association for World Health (AAWH) is the directing organization for World AIDS Day observances in this country. They can provide resource materials and assistance in planning a community remembrance for World AIDS Day, or any other day. They can be reached at 202/466-5883.

*Work within your own organizations*

– – – – – – – – – – –

One of the best ways to advocate for AIDS awareness in your community is through groups you already belong to. Organizations that have stature in the community are often most effective in reaching a broad range of people. Even groups that are not overtly charitable can provide forums for education and can help coordinate other efforts. Members of these organizations can be a great help in drawing on the resources the group has to offer.

People are much more receptive to members of their own groups than they are to strangers. Any group can provide a structure for delivering services, raising funds, sponsoring events, or simply informing members. Deciding what to do is not the hard part. This book is full of suggestions. The challenge is in raising the group's awareness and inspiring its members to take action.

In general, you can take three different approaches in working with organizations:

* ❋ Educate the group about AIDS.
* ❋ Encourage the group to raise money or give time to other organizations that are fighting AIDS.
* ❋ Organize the group to provide services directly.

## GROUP AND ORGANIZATIONAL RESOURCES

A wide variety of groups can provide forums and help in AIDS education and services:

Churches, synagogues, mosques, temples, and other religious groups have excellent resources for reaching people, as well as evoking compassion and good works. Getting involved, or getting your church involved, in the AIDS Interfaith Network can be a great way to promote AIDS awareness. Contact them at 202/546-0807.

Business and professional groups are well-respected in most communities. They can be effective in raising funds directly, or they can simply lend their good names through endorsements or by sponsoring other efforts.

Everyone belongs to informal groups they might take for granted. These informal groups can be just as effective as others. For instance, the crowd in front of the bagel store on weekends or the riders of the 7:25 express train might be receptive to leaflets passed out by a regular attendee.

A number of traditional public service organizations in your community are probably already involved in the fight against AIDS. These include the American Red Cross, National Urban League, National Council of La Raza, Boys' Clubs and Girls' Clubs, the Rotary Club, the YMCA and YWCA, and Planned Parenthood.

Many other groups that might help your cause: unions, country clubs, sports clubs, media groups, service clubs (Elks, Junior League), art and performance groups, and so on.

130 *Advocate for AIDS awareness in the workplace*

Use your skills as an advocate to let your employer and co-workers know that people with HIV or AIDS can continue to be productive and valuable workers. The workplace is one of the most effective and crucial places to raise AIDS awareness.

Many of the most important issues surrounding AIDS are brought out in the workplace. If people with AIDS are able and allowed to work, they will not feel like outcasts or dependents on society. If employers accommodate their work and workplace for employees and customers with AIDS, they are letting them know that they are valuable, important people. The ability to keep working is a vital part of everyone's self-image as a contributor to society.

Every employer also has, or should have, a strong interest in keeping employees educated, safe, and healthy. Preventive measures taken by your employer can dramatically reduce future health care costs and the loss of valuable employees.

Every employer will have to face AIDS. More than two-thirds of all employers of more than 2,500 people and nearly one in ten employers of fewer than 500 people have already had an employee with HIV or AIDS. AIDS has already generated more discrimination lawsuits than any single disease in the history of the United States. People with HIV and AIDS are protected by federal law against discrimination in the workplace just like other employees with disabilities.

The National Leadership Coalition on AIDS (NLCA) is a national group of business and labor leaders working to prevent the spread of HIV through effective workplace AIDS education policies and practices. They can offer you and your employer support in developing such policies in your own workplace. You can reach NLCA at 202/429-0930.

All of the methods for working with groups discussed earlier in this chapter are also effective in the workplace. Here are a few ideas:

✳ MAKE A STATEMENT. Encourage a group from your work to appear together under a banner at a local AIDS event.

✳ INVITE SPEAKERS TO YOUR WORK. Organizations like the National Association of People with AIDS (NAPWA) or the Red Cross can make presentations appropriate to every type of workplace.

✳ HAVE A FOOD DRIVE. People will feel inspired to contribute if everyone else is contributing.

132

✳ VOLUNTEER AS A GROUP. Help out an AIDS service group on certain days of the week with a group of co-workers.

✳ ASK FOR MATCHING FUNDS. Encourage your employer to offer matching funds for employee contributions to AIDS causes.

✳ PROVIDE GOODS AND SERVICES TO AIDS CAUSES. Just as individuals may have special skills and resources to offer, businesses are often uniquely able to give certain items or services. Encourage your workplace to contribute computer time, printing, equipment loans, even leftover food if you work at a bakery or a restaurant. Many of these resources can be of great help, and don't even cost your employer anything extra.

### Make sure your workplace complies with the Americans with Disabilities Act

The Americans with Disabilities Act of 1992 (ADA) requires all employers of more than fifteen people to ensure that they do not discriminate against people with disabilities, including people with HIV and AIDS. Employers must know:

✳ They cannot refuse to hire or promote people because they are infected with HIV.

✳ They cannot require potential or current employees to be tested for HIV unless all employees in the same position are tested and the test is consistent with business necessity. In most cases, testing is not consistent with business necessity.

✻ They must make reasonable accommodations to the work environment or process so that a qualified person can perform essential job functions. This might include allowing time off for medical treatments or building a wheelchair ramp.

✻ They must provide services to HIV-infected people without discrimination.

These are just a few main provisions of the ADA and how they apply to people with AIDS and HIV. For more complete information, contact these organizations:

BUSINESS RESPONDS TO AIDS RESOURCES SERVICE:
800/458-5231 or
800/243-7012 *for TDD service of the hearing impaired*
EQUAL EMPLOYMENT OPPORTUNITY COMMISSION—
ADA HOTLINE:
800/669-EEOC or
800/800-3302 *for TDD service of the hearing impaired*
NATIONAL LEADERSHIP COALITION ON AIDS:
202/429-0930

### *Develop a written policy*

If your employer doesn't have one already, you should encourage him or her to develop an AIDS-in-the-Workplace policy. A clear policy ensures that all employees are treated fairly and consistently. The CDC has a wealth of information and resources to help employers write AIDS-in-the-Workplace policies. They can even supply sample policies.

## LEARNING MORE ABOUT HOW TO INVOLVE YOUR COMMUNITY IN THE FIGHT AGAINST AIDS

### Books about AIDS in the workplace

*AIDS in the Workplace: Legal Questions and Practical Answers* by WILLIAM F. BANTA (Lexington Books, 1993)

*We Are All Living with AIDS: How You Can Set Policies and Guidelines for the Workplace* by EARL C. PIKE (Deaconess Press, 1993)

### Books about community activism

*Fifty Things You Can Do to Fight AIDS* by NEAL HITCHENS (Lowell House, 1992)

*You Can Do Something About AIDS* edited by SASHA ALYSON (a public service project of the publishing industry, 1988)

# Getting Young People Involved

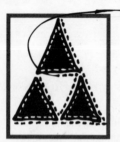 Young people can do more than learn about AIDS—they can be valuable advocates and volunteers in their own right. It's important to involve your children in your efforts. With direct, personal experience, they will learn about the disease and develop an attitude and awareness that can lead to safer choices down the road.

Getting involved in AIDS causes can be a great thing for a family to do together. Families can strengthen their own relationships while they make a huge difference in other people's lives. If you're tired of only doing "fun" things that your children forget about in a few weeks, why not try to involve them in something more meaningful? This chapter will offer ideas about how young people—either on their own or with their families—can get involved in the fight against AIDS. People of all ages have something to give.

138 *Teaching their friends*
- - - - - - - - - -

Young people are very effective at reaching—and teaching—their peers. They can be both advocates and educators. If your children are knowledgeable about HIV and AIDS, they can help encourage awareness and compassion by sharing their knowledge and understanding with others around them.

### Being an AIDS awareness advocate

It's just as important, perhaps more so, for young people to be AIDS awareness advocates as it is for adults. Any informed person who shares knowledge with others or corrects myths and misinformation is an advocate, and young people, just like adults, can help call attention to uninformed or insensitive comments about AIDS.

Many children will respond to the stigmatized nature of the disease and the fact that it involves uncomfortable issues such as sex and sexuality by cracking jokes and making light of it. Calling friends and classmates on this kind of behavior, even asking them where they heard something that isn't true, helps to demystify AIDS and encourage acceptance and understanding.

Being an advocate among rebellious teenagers may be harder than among adults, but it's vitally important. Being an advocate doesn't mean you have to be boring or give unwanted advice. Someone who knows the facts and uses them well will always be respected. Teenagers are much better at reaching each other at this age than they are at taking advice from authority figures.

Vince, a high school junior in Kansas, was worried that his friends would give him a hard time for his stance on AIDS awareness. He says:

*"I was worried they'd think I was weird or something, cause I'd be talking about safe sex. But I don't make too big a deal out of it, just kind of say my piece when it comes up. I think I make a difference."*

*Teaching their peers*

Young people who want to take their advocacy a step further can attend some simple classes and become trained peer counselors. Many high school students have become part of their local peer HIV/AIDS education efforts through their school or local health departments. They are trained in the facts of HIV and AIDS, and they deliver this message to fellow students. A peer education program can train high school students to offer workshops or provide materials about issues such as sexual decision making, communication, and safer sex.

Students seem more willing to accept the teachings of their peers when dealing with sensitive and scary topics such as AIDS. Teneicia, a high school student, was trained in peer education by her local Red Cross. She goes along with Red Cross speakers to schools throughout her district giving workshops on safe sex, "condom sense," and the dangers of injecting drugs. She says:

*"I think I reach the other kids better than older speakers. I feel like I'm doing something really worthwhile, and it looks really good on my college applications."*

For information on peer education efforts in your area, contact your state AIDS office (a state-by-state listing is found at the back of this book).

### *Looking out for each other*

Parents know that there is only so much they can do to protect their children. In most cases, they won't be there to offer advice when it's needed most. That's why its so important for young people, especially

> "Sex now isn't like when our parents were young. They only had to worry about pregnancy. Now we have AIDS to think about. We've got to protect ourselves and help protect each other."— JASON, AGE 20

teenagers, to be willing and able to say the right thing at the right time. Someone needs to be there at parties when friends have had too much to drink and are tempted to have unsafe sex. It's common, responsible behavior to designate a driver to stay sober and make sure everyone makes it home safely. Why not also designate a friend to make sure no one who's been drinking does anything that might lead to risky sexual situations?

142 *Organizing at school*

------------

Schools are a great place for young people to promote AIDS awareness and help those in the community. Schools may already have an AIDS education program in place, but students can supplement these efforts. Its important that AIDS awareness not be perceived as something only adults can teach to young people. Students should play an active role. With so many young, energetic people in one place, schools can also make a difference in the community at large. School organizations can help raise money or even provide AIDS services directly.

### Promote better AIDS education

If there isn't already an AIDS education program at school or the program is inadequate, students can lobby for improvement through the student government, advisory committees, or by circulating petitions.

"The school board and a lot of parents were upset by the idea that the schools were going to teach us how to have sex or that AIDS education would be like basically saying, 'Go for it, kids.' They wanted the school to teach us about abstinence and not even talk about condoms. That's really lame, because if kids are going to have sex, nothing is going to stop them. I know how

## Organize an AIDS awareness day or week    

Organizing an AIDS awareness day or week at school is a great way to bring young people together and focus attention on the problem. Organizations can help provide materials and even speakers at such events, but it's best if students take the initiative. Students can also share their experience as peer counselors or AIDS caregivers.

The CDC can provide materials for young people to distribute at school, clubs, church youth groups or other extracurricular activities. (CDC National AIDS/HIV Hotline, 800/342-2437, twenty-four hours a day.) The National Association of People with AIDS (202/898-0414), can provide speakers and facilitators for assemblies or classes. You might also contact your local AIDS service organization. Many groups maintain lists of speakers and can tailor the speaker for the group, such as sending a teenager to a high school.

important it is to tell the whole story, so kids won't make dumb choices and end up with AIDS. So I went to a school board meeting as the official student representative and explained all this to the group. I think it's really important for them to hear from someone who knows what it's like to be a teenager today." —DONNA, A HIGH SCHOOL JUNIOR

144

"For my citizenship issues class, I passed out red ribbons for AIDS awareness, as well as information cards and brochures, at a local mall and movie theater. I also helped staff a teen hotline to answer questions about HIV and AIDS." —JENNY, AGE 16

### Have a food drive

Students can donate food to a local AIDS service organization. Be sure to check with the organization about what types of food are needed.

### Have a cheaper prom

Students can encourage their schools and classmates to divert funds or scale down special events such as senior proms and use the extra money for AIDS causes.

John, a high school student in southern California, was head of the organizing committee for senior class activities. He says:

*"We usually go to some place like Magic Mountain for 'grad night.' But we wanted to do something different after we went to an AIDS ward for Social Living class. So instead of spending a lot of money for one fun night, we made a donation to a local hospice and volunteered on grad night. I think most of us will remember it a lot longer than a few roller coaster rides."*

### Work with school groups

Any school group can also be a forum for AIDS education or community activism, even the chess club, the French club, the cheerleaders, or the school band. Have the hiking club write letters to a local congressional representative. Donate the ticket sales from the school play to an AIDS cause. The student council can deliver lunches to people with AIDS once a week.

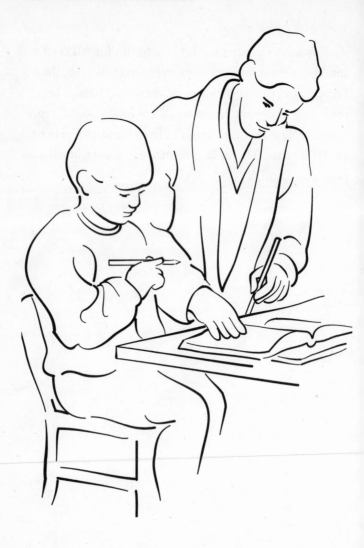

## Becoming junior buddies

- - - - - - - - - - - -

Just as you shouldn't hide your children from people with AIDS, you shouldn't hide people with AIDS from your children. Young people can provide important services and emotional support. People with AIDS often especially appreciate help from children, since many parents don't allow their children near people with AIDS. Children's energy and optimism can be a valuable source of inspiration and hope to people with AIDS. Older children can take some responsibility for providing services themselves, while younger ones can accompany you when you make visits.

Fernando is a sixth-grader who lives near Boston. When Bill, a neighbor with AIDS, got too sick to do his shopping, Fernando's mother asked him to help out and buy things at the store for Bill.

*"At first I was afraid that I could catch it just by breathing around him. I was also afraid of how he'd look but it wasn't a big deal. Then he started talking to me about the Red Sox and we started going to games."*

Now Fernando stops by to see if Bill needs anything whenever he goes to the store. They watch almost every Red Sox game together, and Bill helps Fernando with his English homework.

148

Here are some ideas for how children can help people with AIDS:

* ❋ Helping with yard work, cleaning, and general chores
* ❋ Preparing food and care packages
* ❋ Caring for pets
* ❋ Doing errands

## Raising funds

As anyone who has ever succumbed to a Girl Scout's cookie pitch knows, children make terrific fund-raisers. They can use many of the same tactics used by adults. They can participate in walkathons and bike-athons, sell raffle tickets, or sell tickets to fund-raising events. The United Nations International Children's Emergency Fund (UNICEF) has shown that trick-or-treating at Halloween can also be a good fund-raising opportunity. Neighborhood children can also band together and put on a play, carnival, or talent show to raise money for AIDS. And of course, you can't go wrong with an old-fashioned bake sale or car wash.

# Organizing and participating in group projects

Get the scout troop, church youth group, or just the children in the neighborhood together for some activities that can help raise AIDS awareness in the community.

### Make AIDS Memorial Quilt panels

Young people can work together to create a memorial panel for someone they know—perhaps a teacher—who has died from AIDS or for children in the local hospice who may not have anyone to make a panel for them. This is a wonderful, creative way to teach children about AIDS and about compassion.

The group can present their finished panel at a local display of the quilt or display it at school, the local mall, a bank or business lobby, at church, or in another public venue, to help educate others about the disease.

A group of second-graders in a Minnesota classroom learned about AIDS the hard way: they lost their first-grade teacher to the disease. Paula, their second-grade teacher wanted them to learn about HIV and AIDS and also wanted them to understand their loss. Paula said:

*"We spent a lot of time talking about Mr. Rickman, what they remembered about him, what he taught them,*

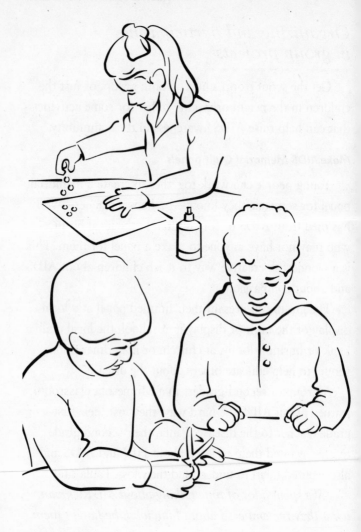

*funny things he would do and say. Then we all made pictures that showed how we felt about him and how much we missed him. We used those pictures as the beginning design for the panel we created for him. Now the panel is completed and is a part of the AIDS Memorial Quilt. I like to think it will help show other kids something about what it's like to lose someone to AIDS."*

### Bring the children on marches

Bring the children along when you go to an AIDS march or vigil. Everyone should know that people fighting AIDS are not just young, single people. Show children that families with other children are involved. It will also be an important bonding event for your family. Your children will gain a strong sense of community responsibility and perhaps find heroes and role models.

**"I lost my brother to AIDS three years ago and I think it's really important for me to be involved in showing people that this can happen to anyone. Hey, it happened to me and I'm a mom in a medium-sized town in the middle of the country. Everyone who dies of AIDS has left people behind who miss them. I like to think that when I bring my toddler to candlelight vigils and marches, I am helping to break down the stereotypes that say this disease only strikes gay people or people who are far away in big cities." —YOLANDA**

152 *Make baby quilts*

Many infants and children are orphaned as a result of the virus and need the love and comfort (and warmth) that a cheerful baby quilt, made by children, can bring. The ABC Quilts organization provides cuddly quilts to babies with AIDS. The quilts are made by volunteers who donate their time, talent, and fabric. Why not have the 4-H club or a school group work together to create these quilts for young people with AIDS?

ABC Quilts has published a book about making these quilts: *Kids Making Quilts for Kids* by ABC Quilts (Quilt Digest Press, 1992).

For more information, contact:

ABC QUILTS
P.O. Box 107
Weatherford, OK 73096

*Draw the faces of AIDS*

Have children make pictures that illustrate what they are learning as part of their AIDS education. Display these art works in schools, malls, business lobbies, and other public spaces as a way of raising AIDS awareness.

# Doing More

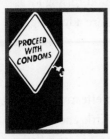

As we have learned, there are many simple and effective ways to help fight AIDS. Perhaps you are already involved and you want to do more. This chapter looks at ways you can become involved at a higher level and build on your commitment to fighting AIDS. Some of the suggestions that follow may not be for everyone, but for those who feel the need to be more active, these methods have been shown to be very effective.

154 *Raise money*

- - - - - - - - - - - -

If you can't spare any money to make donations, use your time, energy, and special skills to raise money from others. Many ways of raising money can be fun. They can get you involved in your community and help you meet new people. There are several specific fund-raising ideas in other chapters of this book, but here are a few suggestions for a general approach.

### Ask your friends to make contributions

This is one of the simplest and most effective ways to raise money. Many people only need a little encouragement or perhaps some basic information to begin showing their financial support. Everyone is inclined to do something if a friend is doing it too, and people have a much harder time refusing friends than they do the senders of anonymous mailings, telephone callers, or canvassers. It's also much easier to give a check to a friend you trust than it is to do your own research on organizations.

Richard, a Chicago resident, calls himself a "shameless fund-raiser" for HIV and AIDS causes. At birthday and holiday time, he asks friends to contribute money to an AIDS service organization in his name, rather than buying him a present.

### Raise funds at work

Send out a memo or message on the electronic mail system if you have one that you are accepting donations for a worthy AIDS organization. A lot of people will make donations if they think all their co-workers are, especially if you take the initiative and handle the details for them.

Lynn, an employee at a large software company in Silicon Valley, sent out an announcement on her electronic mail that she was riding in a bike-athon. *"I was expecting a few responses, but almost everyone in my department sponsored me. I made over $500!"*

### Get business involved

Encourage local businesses to donate a portion of profits during special times. You can also offer the business extra promotion in return.

**"When I found out my company was matching up to $1000, I felt like I had to give. I didn't want the AIDS center to miss out on any potential money."—TOM, FROM ORLANDO**

### Organize events

Anything that people do for fun can be turned into a fund-raising event: dance-athons, walkathons, bike-athons, even marathons.

*Arrange for matching funds*

Encourage your employer or anyone else in a position to do so to match contributions. Matching funds encourage others to give more because they know their donation will be doubled.

## Give money

We've talked about many creative ways to support the fight against AIDS, but let's not forget the basic ones. Every organization involved in the fight against AIDS needs money: AIDS service organizations, educational programs, research institutions, and political groups.

Whether you're giving your own money or money you've raised, no one has an unlimited amount. You want to make sure that your money is going to the right place. With thousands of organizations fighting AIDS across the country and around the world, how do you choose the ones you want to support? It may not be easy.

Opposite is a list of some of the best-known national organizations.

Many other worthy organizations do important work in the fight against AIDS. To find out about more organizations read *How to Find Information About AIDS* by JEFFREY T. HUBER (Harrington Park Press, 1992). You can

AMFAR/American Foundation
 for AIDS Research
1515 Broadway, Suite 3601
New York, NY 10036-8901
212/682-7440

Gay Men's Health Crisis
129 W. 20th Street
New York, NY 10011
212/807-7035

The Names Project Foundation
310 Townsend, Suite 310
San Francisco, CA 94107
415/882-5500

National Association of People
 with AIDS
P.O. Box 18345
Washington, DC 20036
202/898-0414

National Minority AIDS Council
714 G Street SE
Washington, DC 20003
202/544-1076

Pediatric AIDS Foundation
1311 Colorado Avenue
Santa Monica, CA 90404
310/395-9051

People with AIDS Coalition
31 W. 26th Street
New York, NY 10010
212/532-0290

Project Open Hand
2710 17th Street
San Francisco, CA 94110
415/558-0600

Ryan White Foundation
Merchant's Plaza
Suite 1135 East
101 W. Washington Street
Indianapolis, IN 46204
800/444-RYAN
317/261-0086

San Francisco AIDS Foundation
P.O. Box 6182
San Francisco, CA 94101
800/FOR-AIDS

Shanti Project
525 Howard Street
San Francisco, CA 94105
415/777-CARE

also call the CDC Hotline at 800/342-2437 for information on other national groups or your state AIDS office for information on groups in your area (a state-by-state listing is available at the back of this book).

Always learn as much as possible about any organization you are helping. What services do they provide? To whom do they provide them? What type of research do they conduct? What type of political work do they do?

Some people who want to make sure that every penny they give goes to help people with AIDS like to find out what percentage of donations to an organization are used for operating expenses. There are some small groups that operate completely with donated resources and volunteer staff, so they're able to spend almost all donations on goods or services for people with AIDS. Most of these groups provide services that don't involve large operating costs.

Larger organizations that provide specialized services, conduct research, or do political work will have more operating costs and administrative overhead. This doesn't mean that the money these groups spend on staff, administration, and other operating costs is wasted. Large, stable organizations are vitally important to the fight against AIDS, and they do have legitimate operating expenses.

There are large, well-known organizations that do crucial work across the country. There are also small organizations in your community that focus their efforts locally. Where you choose to give your money depends on what is important to you. Perhaps you want your dollars at work for people with AIDS right in your community. Or maybe you would rather send your donation to a national education and prevention effort aimed at young people. Still others might prefer to fund research efforts in hopes of finding a cure.

Aside from donating to national groups, you can start or join local chapters of national organizations. Working with a national organization can help you get resources and attention for your community efforts at a level that might not be possible if you work alone.

### Creative donations

You don't have to give your money to an established organization. There are other creative and unique ways to support the fight against AIDS, such as making donations or in-kind gifts directly to people with AIDS whom you know. Remember, it is tough for people to feel like they are needy, or a charity case, so give money with sensitivity and discretion.

Here are some alternative ideas for making donations:

✻ Purchase blocks of tickets to local events for use by AIDS service groups.

✻ Sponsor members of local AIDS groups to attend conferences and other events.

✻ Send a child with AIDS to camp.

✻ Donate copies of this book or other educational materials to local school or religious groups.

✻ Hire a house cleaner for someone with AIDS.

✻ Have a meal from a nice restaurant delivered to someone with AIDS.

✻ Offer prize money to local young people for drawing the best AIDS awareness poster or writing the best essay on Why I Help in the Fight Against AIDS.

> "When we were in college, my friend Frank and I always used to eat at this little dive on Fifth Street that served the best Kung Pao chicken. When Frank got sick, I tried to think of a way to help out that might cheer him up at the same time. I had the Kung Pao chicken delivered to his house. He called to tell me he loved it and that it brought him right back to those days. We had a good laugh."—NICK IN MINNEAPOLIS

# *Think globally*

- - - - - - - - - -

AIDS has been devastating to some of the poorer nations. Their needs are desperate, and they have difficulty getting support from wealthier nations.

According to the World Health Organization, nine to ten million people worldwide have been infected with HIV. By the year 2000, an estimated thirty to forty million people will be infected, 90 percent of these in developing countries. Sub-Saharan Africa has been the hardest hit, with approximately seven million adults and children infected since the start of the epidemic.

Treatments for AIDS in poorer countries are far below the standards in more affluent nations. In fact, the thrust of treatment and prevention is drastically different. In many less-developed areas, such as the African nations or South America, resources like clean needles are so scarce that medical workers use dirty, possibly HIV-infected needles to administer vitally needed vaccines to the populace. In some of these countries, treatment of AIDS may be only aspirin and bed rest.

The World Health Organization and the Pan-American Health Organization help to provide treatment and education programs in poor countries. Show your support by

162

sending a generous donation earmarked for international
AIDS care and education to:

WORLD HEALTH ORGANIZATION
or
PAN-AMERICAN HEALTH ORGANIZATION
525 23rd Street NW
Washington, DC 20037
202/861-3200

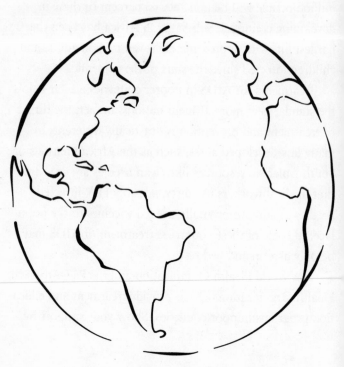

# Get involved in political actions

A big part of the fight against AIDS takes place in the political arena. We can do a lot in our communities, but to really stop AIDS and to work in a coordinated, effective way, we need leadership and support from our government. We must ensure that our local, state, and federal government representatives are fully informed and aware of and responsive to AIDS issues. Some of the most important responsibilities that the government must meet in the fight against AIDS include:

✳ FUNDING RESEARCH into treatments and cures. The federal government is the largest funder of AIDS research through agencies such as the National Institutes of Health (NIH) and the CDC. Obviously, politics plays a big role in determining how much money there is for research, where the money goes, and how it is spent.

✳ PROTECTING INDIVIDUAL CIVIL RIGHTS. The Americans with Disabilities Act, passed in 1992, prohibits discrimination against all disabled Americans, including those with HIV and AIDS.

✳ PROTECTING THE POPULATION. The government is responsible for protecting public health in a number of ways, including the regulation of blood banks to prevent the passing of contaminated blood.

❊ EDUCATING THE PUBLIC. The CDC, the Surgeon General, the White House AIDS czar, and state health departments are all supposed to help educate the public about important health issues.

❊ KEEPING UP WITH NEW DEVELOPMENTS. The government should respond to new HIV-related information and issues and respond appropriately by, for example, mandating the implementation of universal precautions to protect health care providers.

❊ FUNDING HEALTH CARE. All but the richest people with AIDS may end up on Medicaid and disability whether they have insurance or not. Many insurance policies don't provide enough benefits for people with AIDS, particularly if they need several years of care. Dying of AIDS is very expensive. The government makes decisions about the rationing of care through the allotment of funds to these agencies.

How the government carries out these tasks has a far-reaching impact on the quality of life for people with AIDS and for everyone else. Individuals in this society must monitor the government's activities and see that it carries out these important responsibilities in the most effective and compassionate way possible.

## STAY ON TOP OF AIDS LEGISLATION

Find out when important legislation affecting AIDS research, education, treatment, or services is pending in your state legislature or in Washington. You can find out what AIDS legislation is being considered in Washington by reading the AIDS Action Council newsletters.

To subscribe to the AIDS Action Council newsletters contact:

AIDS Action Council
1875 Connecticut Avenue, NW
Suite 700
Washington, DC 20009
202/986-1300

The National Gay and Lesbian Task Force also does AIDS-related lobbying, monitors the progress of AIDS funding bills, and acts as a clearinghouse of information. You can subscribe to their newsletter and AIDS updates by contacting:

National Gay and Lesbian Task
Force
1734 14th Street NW
Washington, DC 20009
202/332-6483

*Write to legislators*

Legislators take letters from their constituents very seriously. In fact, many political analysts and activists believe that one letter from a voter represents the views of at least 100 others. So your single effort is really worth 101 votes to a politician. There's a lot more power in the pen than you may think.

You can also use the newer media such as electronic mail and FAX machines to get your point across. When you write, mention specific legislation. If your legislators have not taken a position on a specific bill or policy, make your opinion clear, and ask them for theirs. Let them know that people do pay attention to their positions on these issues. And don't confine your letters to members of the House and Senate. Write school board members, city council members, the president, your governor, or any other political leaders who might make a difference. Get your friends, family, and co-workers to write on the same topic. Legislators will perceive this is as a groundswell of popular opinion.

To reach your representative in the House, write:

Rep. _____
U.S. House of Representatives
Washington, DC 20515

To reach your senator, write:

Senator _____

U.S. Senate

Washington, DC 20510

### Consider the AIDS voting records of candidates when you vote

Many political leaders believe that if they support AIDS legislation, the public will perceive that they condone premarital sex, homosexuality, drug use, or other practices some consider immoral. Others simply avoid the issue.

It's important to let these leaders know that supporting AIDS legislation does not mean approval of any type of behavior. Tell them that you and your friends and neighbors want this crisis faced with a realistic, pragmatic approach that is not bound by narrow or unrealistic ideology. Tell them you want them to enact programs that will help save lives right now in this world, with all of its imperfections. Let them know that their inaction on this issue will cost them your vote.

Some politicians have actively opposed any compassionate response to the epidemic. They have consistently blocked funding for AIDS research and hindered AIDS education programs because they believe such assistance encourages immorality and that people with AIDS deserve a cruel death. If you are represented by one of these politicians, you should consider contributing your time or money to more compassionate candidates in the next election.

The AIDS Action Council tracks the AIDS voting record of every legislator at both the state and federal levels. To find out where your representatives stand, call 202/986-1300.

## Use your clout as a consumer

You have great power as a consumer. When you purchase a product or use a service provided by a business, you are supporting all of that business's activities, including its AIDS policies. Many businesses have been conscientious citizens and have responded to AIDS with compassion. Some have not taken any position. Others have discriminated against their employees with AIDS, refused to support AIDS services in their communities, and donated to the election campaigns of politicians who oppose funding of AIDS research and services.

It's just as important to inform businesses of your concern with AIDS policy as it is to inform politicians. Large corporations in particular have enormous influence over public policy, the lives of their employees, and the communities where they do business. The list of companies that have no clear AIDS policy and do not actively support any AIDS causes is much longer than the following list of businesses with especially good AIDS policies. Let the other businesses know that as influential citizens, they are obliged to help the communities in which they earn their profits.

### Support AIDS-friendly businesses

The following businesses have been especially compassionate and responsive to the epidemic. Show your support of their policy with your loyal patronage. Write these companies to let them know that their policy is making them money: American Express, Apple Computer, Citibank, Fox, Inc., Home Box Office, IBM, Kellogg's, Levi-Strauss, Pepsico, Seagram Distillers, Showtime Universal Pictures/MCA, Warner Bros., Woolworth, and Xerox.

### Withhold support from AIDS-unfriendly businesses

Some companies have mistreated their employees with AIDS, consistently refused to support AIDS charities, or donated money to the election campaigns of politicians with very irresponsible AIDS policies. Boycotts are in effect against many of these companies' products and services. If you join one of these boycotts, call or write the company to let them know that their policies are costing them money. Contact the AIDS Action Council for information about the AIDS policies of particular companies.

# *Help work for a cure*

- - - - - - - - - - - -

You don't have to be infected with the virus that causes AIDS to participate in studies for AIDS treatments. Researchers need HIV-negative people as members of control groups in many research studies. All potential drugs or vaccines must be tested on both HIV-positive and HIV-negative people. Remember, you need to understand any possible risks and/or benefits of participating in a particular study or research effort.

To find out if studies are being conducted in your area, contact your city or county health department or your local AIDS research organization. For information about clinical trials sponsored by NIH and FDA-approved drug efficacy trials, call 800/TRIALS-A.

# Mourning Those Lost to AIDS

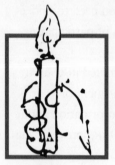

Mourning is the process by which we grieve for the loss of our loved ones, acknowledge their passing, and continue with our lives. If we try to stifle parts of the process—try to avoid grief—we may fail to overcome the loss and begin healing.

Mourning is never easy. When a loved one dies of AIDS, it is still more difficult. Because of the stigma of the disease, you may not be able share your grief readily with those around you. You may also not receive as much support from friends and family as you might when someone dies from a more accepted disease.

Honoring the memory of those who die from AIDS is as important as treating them well when they are alive. Remembering them with love and pride means losing less to the disease. Trying to forget them and ignore or conceal how they died will only make the loss more painful.

174 *Allow yourself to grieve*
------------------------------

The death of a loved one is a great tragedy, no matter how much the dying may exhort us to celebrate their life and not mourn their death. Survivors will always feel a great sense of loss. It's normal during any grieving process to have a number of powerful, debilitating emotions.

The most painful part of the mourning process begins after the formal ceremonies of death are complete. At the time of death and shortly afterward, the process of making arrangements and settling affairs, as well as the added support of friends and family, often make this time more endurable. Longstanding issues and tensions are put aside. The loss is too recent to comprehend. Survivors at this stage often feel a sense of calm and purpose, but after the memorial service, when normal life is supposed to resume, is when the real grief sets in.

Here is a simplified list of the most general feelings experienced by most survivors:

✳ DENIAL AND DISBELIEF. Many survivors cannot believe that death has occurred. They cannot accept that their loved ones—who were so recently talking, laughing, crying—are really gone for good. Many survivors cannot bring themselves to move any of the deceased person's possessions; they talk about the dead as if they were still alive.

✳ DESPAIR. Once survivors acknowledge that a loved one is truly gone, they often feel overwhelming sorrow and a sense that life is not possible without the person who died. They may also feel a sense of personal disintegration—that they cannot function without the support and strength of the one who died and that they are incompetent and weak. This may lead to depression. Those in grief often feel paralyzed, unable to talk or even to move, much less take any initiative or any pleasure in life.

✳ ANGER. Survivors often get very angry at friends, society, or even God, that such a thing can occur and strike down good people.

✳ GUILT. Caregivers and parents especially often feel guilty that they could not prevent this from happening, that if they had somehow provided some special type of care, their loved ones might have been cured, or at least might have lived longer and died with less pain. They may also feel guilty that they are alive and did not suffer as much as their loved one did. As the mourning process continues, they may even feel guilty about beginning to take pleasure in life again—feel that this somehow betrays the memory of their dead loved one.

All of these emotions are common to every mourning process. Certain aspects of dying from AIDS, however, make the grief more acute and mourning more difficult:

✳ MULTIPLE LOSSES. In some communities, survivors must cope with the loss of several friends and loved ones over the course of a few years. This is the single biggest difference between an AIDS death and the death of a loved one from any other cause. When someone dies of cancer or gets hit by a car, it's an isolated incident that is not likely to be repeated in a family or a community. But AIDS deaths are part of an ongoing succession of deaths, with dozens of friends, family members, and lovers all dying. Only the losses faced in wartimes are comparable.

✳ PREMATURE LOSS. Death seems natural in old age. Parents expect to die before their children. So when a young person dies, the loss is premature and thus seems more grievous.

✳ STIGMA. Fearing the scorn of others, families may try to hide the cause of a loved one's death or even the death itself.

✳ LACK OF FAMILY SUPPORT. Many who die from AIDS, as well as their survivors, are alienated from or ostracized by their families, so they don't receive the invaluable support of their family of origin.

✳ EXTREME SUFFERING. Death from AIDS often involves a long process of deterioration and acute suffering, making the survivors feel more pain in empathy.

✳ No legal recognition of relationships.
Because of the lack of legal recognition of gay relationships, partners of those who have died from AIDS may
not even be allowed time off from work to mourn.
They may also have property disputes with family members of the deceased, who may refuse to acknowledge the
relationship.

✳ Loneliness. Those who have been the primary
caregiver for someone with AIDS may find that their
other relationships have deteriorated while they were cen-
tering their lives around caring for their dying loved one.

✳ Fear for one's own health. If the mourner was
intimate with the person who died, he or she may also
carry HIV and face the prospect of deteriorating and
dying without the support of a partner.

Survivors sometimes hold onto the memory of their
lost loved ones to an unhealthy degree, refusing to disturb
any of their things or holding conversations with the
deceased several months—even years—after their death.
Others feel they can't cope without the consistent, self-
destructive use of drugs or alcohol. But, not allowing for
grief and not accepting the separation of death can prevent people from reconstructing their lives. It is important
to find a middle ground between trying to forget or
ignore the painful loss and obsessively clinging to it.

*Working through grief*

-- -- -- -- -- -- -- -- -- --

Allowing yourself to grieve does not mean that you must do it alone. You should get help if possible. There are a number of ways to get support during the grieving process. Some of them are listed here. Seek them out. Only by reaching out to others and allowing new people into your life can you gradually come to accept your loss and rebuild your hope for the future. Here are several possibilities:

### Reach out to friends and loved ones

When dealing with the death of a loved one, people often tend to fall into isolation. Stay in touch with everyone you know and reestablish contact with good friends with whom you may have lost touch. It's important that you not be alone all the time.

### Seek therapy and counseling

Professional counselors or therapists can be of enormous help to those in mourning. Survivors often fall into self-destructive patterns or fail to observe their own behavior objectively. Professional counselors who have worked with many people in mourning can recognize normal and abnormal grieving processes and can help you get back on track. You don't have to have acute symptoms or be "crazy" to go for counseling. Mourning is a very difficult process, and many of the institutions that used to help people through it, such as the church and the family, are not available for everyone today.

For referrals to counselors and mental health professionals in your area, contact your state or local mental health office or the council on mental health in your area.

## Attend grief support groups

Support groups are important at every stage in the disease process; they are especially valuable during mourning. Sharing your grief with others who have faced a similar loss will help to make you feel less alone. There are support groups for those who have lost someone to AIDS in most communities. Many survivors build valuable, long-lasting relationships in these groups. To find an AIDS survivors support group or bereavement group in your area, contact your local AIDS service organization.

## Make a quilt panel

Make a panel for the AIDS Memorial Quilt to remember the life of your friend or loved one lost to AIDS. Each three-by-six-foot panel in the quilt is a tribute to someone lost to AIDS. You don't have to be an expert at sewing or crafts to design and create a panel. You may want to collaborate with friends and loved ones who also want to share their memories. Remember to include the full name of the person you are making the panel for on the panel, as well as additional information such as birth and death dates. You can also include images of the person's favorite things, hobbies, pets, and so on. Make your panel durable; it will be sewn into a twelve-by-twelve-foot square along with seven other panels and then folded and refolded as it is sent to displays around the world.

For more information and assistance contact the NAMES PROJECT FOUNDATION at 415/882-5500.

### Go to a Quilt display

A display of the AIDS Memorial Quilt brings together people from all parts of the community to grieve, to hope, and to simply acknowledge the scope of the epidemic. The quilt plainly shows the enormity of the loss to AIDS, but it just as powerfully evokes the strength, hope, and sheer vitality of the survivors. It is as much a monument to the survivors of AIDS as a memorial to those lost. No one leaves a display without feeling somehow changed. For those in mourning, this change is very positive and healing.

For more information about quilt displays in your area, contact the NAMES PROJECT FOUNDATION.

### Attend a candlelight vigil

Like displays of the quilt, candlelight vigils and other types of public mourning ceremonies provide opportunities for people in mourning to grieve together, to remember, to celebrate and to renew themselves.

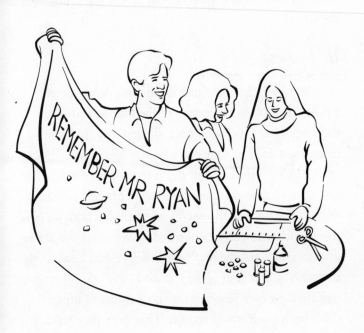

*Seek spiritual solace*

Attending religious services or doing any type of spiritual activity can help you draw strength from others and see beyond your immediate troubles. Even if you haven't participated in any spiritual activities for years, or have never done so, you may find them reassuring and inspiring in this time of crisis. Any activity from reading books on meditation to attending church services may help to inspire you.

## *Be honest*

Don't keep the cause of a loved one's death secret. Cover-ups prolong the stigma of the disease and shame the memory of those who have already died. In some cases, the family of someone who has died from AIDS wishes to keep the cause of death secret because they fear the scorn of their communities or other family members. But in the long run, this secret accomplishes nothing positive. Those who keep it often end up resenting those who do not. Don't assume that people will respond negatively to knowing that your loved one died of AIDS. Allow them to have their own responses without trying to protect them from the truth. If you don't like how they react, you have the opportunity to do a little consciousness-raising.

# Learning more about mourning those lost to AIDS

### Books about loss and grief

*Beyond Grief: A Guide for Recovering from the Death of a Loved One* by Carol Staudacher (New Harbinger, 1987)

*Death, the Final Stage of Growth* by Elisabeth Kübler-Ross (Touchstone, 1975)

*The Grief Recovery Handbook: A Step-by-Step Program for Moving Beyond Loss* by John W. James and Frank Cherry (Harper and Row, 1988)

*Healing Our Losses: A Journal for Working Through Your Grief* by Jack Miller (Resource, 1993)

*On Death and Dying* by Elisabeth Kübler-Ross (Collier, 1969)

# How to Call an AIDS Hotline, State by State

Alabama   800/228-0469

Alaska   800/478-2437

Arizona   800/265-3300

Arkansas   800/448-8305

Northern California
   800/347-2437

Southern California
   800/922-2437

Colorado   800/252-2437

Connecticut   800/342-2437

Delaware   800/422-0429

District of Columbia
   202/332-2437

Florida   800/352-2437

Georgia   800/551-2728

Hawaii   800/922-1313

Idaho   208/345-2277

Illinois   800/243-2437

Indiana   800/848-2437

Iowa   800/445-2437

Kansas   800/232-0040

Kentucky   800/654-2437

Louisiana   800/922-4379

Maine   800/851-2437

Maryland   800/638-6252

Massachusetts   800/235-2331

Michigan   800/872-2437

Minnesota   800/248-2437

Mississippi   800/537-0851

Missouri   800/522-2437

Montana   800 /233-6668

Nebraska   800 /782-2437

Nevada   800 /842-2437

New Hampshire   800 /872-8909

New Jersey   800 /624-2377

New Mexico   800 /545-2437

New York   800 /541-2437

North Carolina   800 /342-2437

North Dakota   800 /472-2180

Ohio   800 /332-2437

Oklahoma   800 /535-2437

Oregon   800 /777-2437

Pennsylvania   800 /662-6080

Puerto Rico   809 /765-1010

Rhode Island   800 /726-3010

South Carolina   800 /322-2437

South Dakota   800 /592-1861

Tennessee   800 /525-2437

Texas   800 /299-2437

Utah   800 /366-2437

Vermont   800 /882-2437

Virginia   800 /533-4138

Virgin Islands   809 /773-2437

Washington   800 /272-2437

West Virginia   800 /642-8244

Wisconsin   800 /334-2437

Wyoming   800/327-2437

# Where to Find HIV/AIDS Organizations

### National and local HIV/AIDS organizations

AIDS NATIONAL INTERFAITH NETWORK
300 I Street NE, Suite 400
Washington, DC 20002
202/546-0807
800 /448-5231 *for a resource guide on issues
related to HIV/AIDS and the religious community*

AMFAR/AMERICAN FOUNDATION FOR AIDS RESEARCH
1515 Broadway, Suite 3601
New York, NY 10036-8901
212/682-7440

ARTHUR ASHE FOUNDATION
100 Park Avenue
New York, NY 10017
212/922-0096

BROADWAY CARES/EQUITY FIGHTS AIDS
165 West 46th, Suite 1300
New York, NY 10036
212/840-0770

BUSINESS RESPONDS TO AIDS RESOURCES SERVICE
800/458-5231
or 800 /243-7012 *for TDD service of the hearing impaired*

CDC/CENTERS FOR DISEASE CONTROL AND PREVENTION
National AIDS Clearinghouse
800 /458-5231

CDC NATIONAL AIDS/HIV HOTLINE
800 /342-2437

DESIGN INDUSTRIES FOUNDATION FOR AIDS (DIFFA)
150 West 26th Street, Suite 602
New York, NY 10001
212/727-3100

EEOC/EQUAL EMPLOYMENT OPPORTUNITY COMMISSION—
ADA HOTLINE:
800 /669-EEOC
800/800-3302 *for TDD service of the hearing impaired*

ELTON JOHN AIDS FOUNDATION
P.O. Box 52066
Atlanta, GA 30355
800 /373-4572

FAMILY AIDS NETWORK
678 Front Street NW, Suite 260
Grand Rapids, MI 49504
616/451-8880

GAY MEN'S HEALTH CRISIS
129 W. 20th Street
New York, NY 10011
212/807-7035

THE MAGIC JOHNSON FOUNDATION
1888 Century Park East, Suite 310
Los Angeles, CA 90067
310/785-0201

THE NAMES PROJECT FOUNDATION
(sponsor of the AIDS Memorial Quilt)
310 Townsend, Suite 310
San Francisco, CA 94107
415/882-5500

NATIONAL ASSOCIATION OF PEOPLE WITH AIDS
P.O. Box 18345
Washington, DC 20036
202/898-0414
202/789-2222 *for information about NAPWA's fax-on-demand
information for people with HIV/AIDS and their caregivers*

NATIONAL COMMUNITY AIDS PARTNERSHIP
1140 Connecticut Avenue NW, Suite 901
Washington, DC 20036
202/429-2820

NATIONAL GAY AND LESBIAN TASK FORCE
1734 14th Street NW
Washington, DC 20009
202/332-6483

NATIONAL LEADERSHIP COALITION ON AIDS
1730 M Street NW, Suite 905
Washington, DC 20036
202/429-0930

NATIONAL MINORITY AIDS COUNCIL
714 G Street SE
Washington, DC 20003
202/544-1076

PAN-AMERICAN HEALTH ORGANIZATION
525 23rd St. NW
Washington, DC 20037
202/861-3200

PEDIATRIC AIDS FOUNDATION
1311 Colorado Ave.
Santa Monica, CA 90404
310/395-9051

PEOPLE WITH AIDS COALITION
31 W. 26th Street
New York, NY 10010
212/532-0290

PROJECT OPEN HAND
2710 17th Street
San Francisco, CA 94110
415/558-0600

RYAN WHITE FOUNDATION
Merchants Plaza, Suite 1135 East
101 W. Washington Street
Indianapolis, IN 46204
800 /444-RYAN, 317/261-0086

SAN FRANCISCO AIDS FOUNDATION
P.O. Box 6182
San Francisco, CA 94101
800/FOR-AIDS

SHANTI PROJECT
525 Howard Street
San Francisco, CA 94105
415/777-CARE

WORLD HEALTH ORGANIZATION
525 23rd Street NW
Washington, DC 20037
202/861-3200

### For written HIV and AIDS materials that can be used in AIDS advocacy, contact:

CENTER FOR HEALTH INFORMATION
P.O. Box 4636
Foster City, CA 94404
415/345-6669

DEPARTMENT OF HEALTH EDUCATION
SIECUS/New York University
Dept. BHG
32 Washington Place
New York, NY 10003

IMPACT AIDS INC.
3692 18th Street
San Francisco, CA 94110
415/861-3397

*For information on AIDS policy and legislation, contact:*

AIDS ACTION COUNCIL
1875 Connecticut Avenue NW, Suite 700
Washington, DC 20009
202/986-1300

CENTER FOR WOMEN POLICY STUDIES
National Resource on Women and AIDS
2000 P Street, Suite 508
Washington, DC 20036
202/872-1770

INTERGOVERNMENTAL HEALTH POLICY PROJECT (IHPP)
AIDS Policy Center
George Washington University
2000 P Street, Suite 800
Washington, DC 20036
202/872-1445

*For help in working with your school board, contact:*

THE AMERICAN CIVIL LIBERTIES UNION
212/944-9800

THE LAMBDA LEGAL DEFENSE AND EDUCATION FUND
212/995-8585

NATIONAL EDUCATION ASSOCIATION
1201 16th Street NW
Washington, DC 20036
202/833-4000

NATIONAL SCHOOL BOARDS ASSOCIATION
1680 Duke Street
Alexandria, VA 22314
703/838-6756

### For information about clinical trials, contact:

800 / TRIALS-A

PROJECT INFORM
1965 Market Street, Suite 220
San Francisco, CA 94103
800/334-7422 *(CA Hotline)*
800/822-7422 *(National Hotline)*

### To reach your congressperson, write to:

Rep. _____

U.S. House of Representatives

Washington, DC 20515

### For your senator, write to:

Senator _____

U.S. Senate

Washington, DC 20510

# The Authors

ANNE GARWOOD is the Panelmaker Relations Coordinator at The NAMES Project Foundation, sponsor of the AIDS Memorial Quilt. As a member of the Development department, she designs and implements programs for panelmaker and donor relations. Based in San Francisco, she works with people from all over the country whose lives have been touched by AIDS, offering support, assistance, and ideas on ways to make a difference in their communities. She has a degree in psychology and human services from the College of St. Mary, Lincoln, Nebraska.

BEN MELNICK is a technical writer at Claris (a subsidiary of Apple Computer) in Santa Clara, California. He won the Northern California Society of Technical Communicators Award of Excellence in 1990 and 1991. Melnick graduated from UC Berkeley with a degree in history.